GLOBETROTTING WITH DISABLED DON

From Cannes to the Caribbean with wheelchairs and walking sticks

Dawn Fallon

Dawn Fallon

Copyright © 2024 Dawn Fallon

Disclaimer

The events described in this book are all true.
I have recreated the events and conversations from my vivid memories
of them, as well as from my travel notes, photograph albums, and travel
diaries.
In some instances, I have changed the names of individuals and places to
maintain their anonymity.

CONTENTS

FOREWORD

"Getting there the hard way…"

Most of us would find lengthy trips exploring Europe quite a challenge. How about doing it with a chap in a wheelchair, his best friend who's had a serious stroke, a four-year-old and his 89-year-old grandfather, endless disability aids plus three of everything for a relaxing day on the beach? Nothing daunts Don who has spina bifida, his wife Dawn and (frequently bemused) youngster Tim as they embark on numerous adventures with friend Geoff. They enjoy the French Riviera with its fabulous dining and dodgy hotels, art galleries, Italy, the majestic Alps (when the mist gives way), markets in Provence, boat excursions, train trips and days (or rather minutes…) on the beach.

Hilarious, humbling and heartwarming, the family's trials and tribulations will make you laugh out loud. Its "I can do this" attitude puts most of us to shame and frankly, there's just no stopping them despite mishaps and accidents galore, all washed down with copious cocktails. Most of us would balk at such experiences but to this extraordinary couple, it's just a matter of… "Getting there the hard way."

Don and Dawn live in Torquay and Don is an enthusiastic member of Dart Sailability where he is a regular and enthusiastic sailor. Dawn has kindly agreed to donate ten per cent of book proceeds to the charity at www.dartsailability.org.

Kate Graeme-Cook
(Trustee and Fundraiser for Dart Sailability)

PART ONE - FRANCE 1999

1. MISHAPS AND MAYHEM

'You're driving on the wrong side of the road!' screams Geoff, after I make a sharp right turn onto a bustling boulevard in Cannes.

My heart races as his panic-stricken words sink in.

Am I?

Oh crikey, I am!

I have just seconds to manoeuvre my way out of imminent danger, avoiding a head-on collision with an oncoming car while dodging a massive truck to my right.

I pull it off, but not without a deafening SMACK! The passenger wing mirror of our hire car shatters as the tail end of the truck catches it.

The truck trundles along without a care in the world. I flash my lights at the driver, but get two squirts of water on the windscreen instead. Undeterred, I keep calm and carry on, pretending nothing has happened.

I'm in Provence with my husband Don, our young son Tim, and a family friend, Geoff.

Don has had a disability since birth—he was born with spina bifida (Lipomyelomeningocele).

Geoff also has a disability—he suffered a stroke twenty years ago.

Tim is four years old.

This is our first trip abroad as a family. Don has never travelled overseas before because he will not fly, and he's only ever had holidays in the UK.

We had planned that Don would do all the driving in our specially adapted Daewoo estate car fitted with hand controls. The spina bifida has caused paralysis in Don's legs and feet and he can't use the pedals, so the hand controls enable him to accelerate or brake using a lever with his right hand.

But the reason I'm driving a hire car is that our Daewoo had a bit of a mishap...

2. HAIRPIN BENDS

It's the 10th of June 1999 and the day starts well with Geoff suggesting we simply must drive up the Col de la Lombarde.

'It's absolutely stunning up there. The views are breathtaking,' Geoff assures us. As he speaks, certain words and syllables get blurted out louder than others in his effort to enunciate them because the stroke has affected Geoff's speech, but he'd been very disciplined with his speech therapy and he's easy to understand.

Despite his disability, Geoff is a well-seasoned traveller. He has been to France many times before to visit his daughter who lives there. Even though Geoff's wife left him after his stroke when he was 50, he has maintained his independence by living alone, doing his own shopping, and cooking for himself. He might be 70, but he lives life to the full.

As I munch on my croissant over breakfast in the villa where we are staying, I look up the Col de la Lombarde in our guidebook and learn that it's a mountain road pass some 2300 metres in altitude on the border between France and Italy overlooking the famous ski resort of Isola 2000.

Adorned with lush greenery, the Col de la Lombarde gracefully links the serene Tinée Valley in the Alpes-Maritimes to the picturesque Stura di Demonte Valley in Piedmont, Italy. Standing at the cusp of the Italian border fills me with a tantalising sense of allure—I could step over it and say I'd been to Italy as well as France.

So off we trek up into the mountains in our Daewoo estate car, with Don behind the wheel. But he's not enjoying the drive along the narrow winding roads at all. He's afraid of heights and feels funny in his tummy.

As we ascend, the mist descends—not part of the plan. We reach the summit, nestled on the Italian border, only to find our anticipation dashed. There's no breathtaking view to greet us.

It's cold.

It's misty.

It's grey.

It's eerie, like a scene straight out of the haunting tale of *The Hound of the Baskervilles*. The air hangs heavy with dampness, chilling us to the bone.

I step over the border to Italy, taking a long whiff of the earthy scent that surrounds me. Then I step back into France.

Undeterred by the gloom, we make the most of it and gather in the warmth of the car to eat our picnic lunch. At this moment, we could be savouring each bite on a foggy day up the Lickey Hills in Birmingham.

Geoff's disappointment is palpable.

'I should have checked the weather forecast,' he bemoans. *Never mind, Geoff. It was a good idea.*

The experience triggers thoughts about national borders. Such fragile things, I ponder, as I consider our elderly friend in Hungary—she's lived in three different countries over the past 70 years without moving house.

As we make our way back down, we arrive at the skiing village of Isola, only to find it eerily desolate. *Isola by name and isolated by nature* comes to mind, as the village itself bears its name and reflects its nature. In June, it exudes an overwhelming sense of melancholy. I close my eyes, attempting to envision the bustling atmosphere of the skiing season, filled with the laughter of bobble-hatted skiers tucking into their tapas and colourful cocktails, against a spectacular snowy backdrop. But the early summer landscape offers nothing to behold. It remains a solitary and forsaken place, leaving me with a profound feeling of loneliness and abandonment.

We continue downhill, the road curving sharply with each hairpin bend and perilous cliff edge. Our stomachs churn uneasily—a queasy sensation intensifying with every twist and turn. We pass random signs displaying vivid images of rocks cascading down the mountainside, serving as a stark reminder of the lurking danger. The thought of a rock crashing onto our windscreen sends shivers down our spines.

Then, just as Don navigates a treacherously tight bend, there it is...

3. UNE GRANDE PIERRE

A large stone had fallen slap-bang in the middle of the road.

Don has seconds to act. He can't go around the stone as the road isn't wide enough, so he has to choose whether to do an emergency stop or drive on and hope the car glides over it. Indecisive, he combines both (a bad idea) and hits the stone.

I step out of the car, followed closely by my inquisitive four-year-old, Tim, to inspect the outcome and we see a stream of red fluid flowing like blood down the road. The abrupt halt of the vehicle had brought the front of the car down over the stone, damaging the hydraulic system. We wouldn't be going anywhere. For a long time.

I'm surprisingly calm.

Don is quiet.

Tim is curious.

Geoff busts into tears.

'Oh, oh, oh...I'm sorry for crying. It's the stroke!' he wails. 'I can't help it. I want my mummy!' he bawls.

The unfortunate situation sparks Geoff's sensitive emotions, which are more vulnerable since the stroke. I'd seen him cry before when he'd visited us in Brixham. We live quite close to the Dartmouth Steam Railway and when the steam train sounded off its jaunty whistle as it chug chug chugged itself along Goodrington, it triggered a trickle of tears down Geoff's cheeks. But they were tears of joy, because for Geoff, a former engineer, the thought of a steam engine sent him into paroxysms of happiness. However, these tears stem from anxiety over the accident.

'Now what do we do?' I ask Don just as a car pulls up in front of us. A French couple driving in the opposite direction can see our predicament and give me a lift to the nearest mountain *mairie* (town hall) at Saint-Étienne-de-Tinée where there's a telephone. Not one of us possesses a cell phone—they are still something of a novelty.

Clutching our insurance details, and mighty relieved for the help these kind strangers are giving us, I go into the *mairie.*

'Er... *parlez vous anglais*?' I ask the *mairie* clerk, conscious that I haven't spoken French for almost 25 years.

'*Un peu,*' she responds.

'We were driving down the mountain and we hit a large stone on the road. It's damaged our car and it won't drive.'

'Ah *oui, un moment*, I will ring ze garage.'

She picks up the phone and describes to someone at the other end what has happened in rapid French. I can't understand a word she is saying as my 'O' Level French deserts me. She could have been telling the garage that she'd got an idiot of an English woman feigning trouble and trying to cadge a lift for all I knew. But then I hear three words I recognise: "*une grande pierre.*"

'*Oui! Oui!*' I affirm with enthusiasm, '*Une grande pierre!*' I repeat, gesturing with my hands the size of the stone in the road as I latch on to the words I understand. The clerk looks up at me, nods and smiles—though if I'd have been in her shoes, I'd probably be thinking, "Darn foreigners!"

The French couple give me a lift back to our wounded vehicle, and it's not long before two men come and tow it away to Garage Latil in Étienne-de-Tinée. They are the owners of the garage, a father and son, and they spend two hours working on our car, trying to repair the hydraulic system. We are so grateful for their kindness. I doubt many English garage owners would spend two hours of their time trying to fix a car, and not charge a penny (or a franc) for it. We'd never encountered such kindness from business people anywhere.

But all their work is to no avail - the damage is too severe and we have to contact AA 5-Star to sort out the problem. It was a good thing Don didn't scrimp and scrape trying to save money on our travel insurance as we'd have been completely up the spout if he'd gone with a cheaper option. And AA 5-Star proves indeed to be five-star in every way—they are excellent and say they'll fly us home and ship our car over later...*Ooh, that will be wonderful, and Don will HAVE to fly after all!*

But Don isn't having any of it and insists that they repair our car within the next ten days while we are in France.

They send a taxi to collect us from Garage Latil in Étienne-de-Tinée. Tim at least thinks it's all great fun and enjoys the drama.

We pile into the taxi. Geoff is now calmer and has accepted the situation, but the journey back to our villa is not what we are expecting.

4. LE TAXI

Flying home would have been far safer than the taxi ride back to our villa. *Le chauffeur de taxi* (aka the taxi driver) zips along at a speed which renders us speechless, apart that is from a few tentative words to the taxi driver from Don.

'Er, *parlez-vous Anglais*?' he murmurs to the driver (it's the only French Don knows).

'*Un peu*,' responds the driver, along with a gesticulation of the forefinger and thumb close together.

'Er...do you think it might be best to drive with both hands on the steering wheel, please?' Don requests politely as the driver casually adjusts the steering wheel with the forefinger of his left hand, while his other hand rests on the gear stick.

The perky taxi driver smiles and nods in agreement, disregarding Don's desperate plea as we speed along the road at nearly 100km per hour - a road which displays a chilling statistic (both in French and English) of how many deaths there have been in the past year. Fear grips us, freezing us in our seats. We are petrified.

We make it back to the villa safe and sound, if a little shaken, and spend the next morning quietly at the villa. Then, after lunch, we leave Geoff to have his afternoon nap while Don and Tim accompany me to pick up the hire car from a company called Sixt in St Tropez. We are driven there by another crazy taxi driver who drives just as fast and spends most of the journey chatting on his natty Nokia mobile phone.

The hire car is a whopper and, of course, it's a left-hand drive. It is indeed AA 5-Star luxury—a brand new Volvo, but she is HUGE. I've never driven a left-hand drive car, let alone driven on the right-hand side of the road, but I do not flinch. *I can do this,* is my attitude.

Having wheels again, and not being content with one disaster up the Alps, on the 12th of June we set off again up the mountains to the Cascades du Saut du Loup near Gourdon. It's a fine, cloudless day, and Geoff insists we see more of the Alps. He's certainly a sprightly 70-year-old, full of the love of life.

With utmost certainty, he promises The Cascades will present an awe-inspiring spectacle of the Loup River and its majestic waterfalls. Indeed, they deliver. The scenery is resplendent with the cascading water pooling into emerald-coloured ponds, and the soothing sound of rushing water arrests our ears. The fresh scent of nature surrounds us, creating a truly unforgettable experience. *Thank you, Geoff.*

It's while travelling back to our villa from Gourdon via Cannes that I end up driving on the wrong side of the road with Geoff screaming at me. It's a close shave—especially for Geoff sitting in the front passenger seat as the wing mirror on his side gets shattered. He pulls his right shoulder inwards as if that will shrink the car.

My stupefied passengers are silent as we trundle back to the villa. I would be driving this thing for another ten days. Will I be able to do it without further incident?

5. FROM THE ENGLISH RIVIERA TO THE FRENCH RIVIERA

The reason we've travelled to France with our friend Geoff is that his daughter, Erica, is a villa *gardien* (caretaker) in Provence. She'd left the UK with her partner, Matt, several years before when the negative equity property crisis kicked in during the early 90s. They'd lost their home. So they moved to France and found work looking after the holiday-home villas and swanky boats of wealthy Brits in Provence.

One of her clients is her uncle, who agreed that we would be welcome to stay in his villa free of charge. Geoff, who would normally fly out to France alone, has stayed there many times before, so this is a joint arrangement: he gets to travel with us and we get to stay with him in the villa. *Splendid!*

And that's just how it starts for us…

Travelling to France begins on the 2nd of June 1999 with our Daewoo estate car packed to the gunwales with all our stuff.

Our home in Brixham is on the English Riviera, and after picking up Geoff from his home in Dorset, we set off to the French Riviera. So with Geoff ensconced in the front passenger seat, Don driving, and me and Tim squashed in the back with heaps of baggage between us, we head to Poole for the car ferry. Tim plays peek-a-boo with me around all the gear piled amidst our seats. Geoff is not happy about the luggage situation: one emergency stop and the whole lot would go flying through the windscreen. Being an engineer by trade, Geoff has a keen understanding of velocity, but Don and I are NOT light travellers.

We catch the ferry (the *BarFleur*) at 12.30 p.m. from Poole where Jo, Geoff's favourite lady friend, waves us off and after a pleasant crossing, we arrive in Cherbourg at 6.45 p.m. French time. After a two-hour drive, we arrive at the Hotel Campanile in Lisieux, which Geoff has pre-booked for us, and we round off the day enjoying a pleasant meal with a regional French twist. Then, after a long day of travelling, we sleep well.

The next morning we savour a leisurely all-you-can-eat French-style breakfast and then head to Paris (via Evreux) for the car train. Geoff has cleverly arranged for us to spend a whole day in the City of Light.

'I wonder if any of us will succumb to the Paris Syndrome?' Don queries.

'What's that?' I probe.

'Apparently, it's a sudden onset of culture shock which can make tourists feel very peculiar.'

'You're joking!' I quip.

'No, it's a genuine issue for some visitors to Paris,' Don confirms.

Little do we know that Don will get into a spot of bother and the guards have to step in.

6. UNDER PARIS SKIES

As we approach Paris to find Hotel Campanile near Bercy, we have to enter the *Périphérique* (the French equivalent of the M25 that goes around the capital city).

Geoff loves maps. He might have a physical disability, but his mind is as sharp as a pin and he's a meticulous map reader. He has earmarked the exit we need which will take us into the heart of Paris to our Campanile and he's our navigator.

We find ourselves stuck in bumper-to-bumper traffic on the *Périphérique* (also known as the *Périph*), constantly stopping and starting until we reach our exit. All the while I have an earworm replaying Raymond Froggatt's 1968 hit song "Callow La Vita" with its wistful reference to a Paris park; besides, Raymond is my cousin, so it's extra poignant.

Then Don gets a different earworm and begins humming Edith Piaff's song *"Sous le Ciel de Paris"* (Under Paris Skies). He's clueless about the lyrics so just keeps humming the tune.

'What *is* it that makes French music sound so French?' I ask Don.

'Hmm...I'm not sure. It always has that romantic yearning feeling in it somehow,' he proffers.

'Well, I studied French music for my dissertation and I never really did find out what its elusive quality is, but I think it's something to do with how French composers make use of the major 7th interval in music, creating sexy scrunchy chords, with that longing feeling in a melody. Mind you, I was still none the wiser after I'd studied it, to be honest,' I admit, looking out of the window at the concrete walls of the *Périph.*

'It has that certain *je ne sais quoi* as they say in France,' chimes in Geoff with his wisdom.

Yes, that's it! French music has an intangible quality that makes it so elusively unique.

We exit the *Périph* and pick up speed, but before long we see signs for Paris-Orly airport.

'That's not right,' Geoff announces. 'We're going in the wrong direction!'

Annoyed at being outwitted by the *Périphérique* and that we're now lost and driving *away* from the city centre, Geoff studies the map and sees that there are two rings on the *Périph* - an outer ring and an inner ring. He deduces that we'd got onto the wrong ring when we'd entered it. There's no alternative but to re-enter the *Périph*, by which time the rush hour has started.

After much faffing and fluffing around, we eventually exit *into* the city centre, arriving at Hotel Campanile. By now I have two earworms going around my head—a fusion of both songs merging into one about Paris, and I have a mild headache.

We have the evening free, so we venture to *Gare de Lyon* and find a restaurant to savour a meal in the City of Light. Plus there's no rail fare to pay due to an industrial dispute over safety issues (well done to the French for sticking up for their rights).

We find a classic French restaurant serving traditional local cuisine, and as we tuck into our delicious meals, we can't help but notice Geoff's chicken looks rather pink and somewhat undercooked.

'Are you quite sure you should eat that, Geoff?' asks Don, who is very fussy about eating any type of food with blood in it. Geoff gives him a look of disdain and doesn't flinch as he eats his meal with aplomb. We are a tad concerned he might die from food poisoning.

Early on the morning of the 4th of June, the sky is overcast, but it's mild. Geoff is still alive and well, and we all eat a hearty French breakfast. We deposit our Daewoo estate car at La Bercy station for the overnight *couchette* sleeper train. This train will take us, and our vehicle, to Provence while we sleep onboard later that night. *Bliss!*

We have the entire day to immerse ourselves in the beauty of Paris and make the most of our time, taking in as much as we can of the vibrant energy of the city. Passing by the magnificent Notre Dame Cathedral, the church bells resonated in the air with *sonneries* announcing the services.

We stroll across the River Seine, its sparkling waters reflecting the silver sky, Don in his callipers with walking sticks, and Geoff also with a walking stick, each with their individual and peculiar gait.

I had thought that having Geoff with us would hold us back because of the stroke affecting his left side, but not a bit of it. I'm surprised to discover that once he gains momentum, he can walk as well as anyone. Going up hills is a challenge for him, so he zig-zags it and then it's no problem at all. It's stopping and starting that Geoff finds physically exhausting, but his experience as an engineer gives him the confidence that once his body is in motion, and he gets into a walking rhythm using his stick, he is safe and can get a wriggle on.

Don's disability also affects mobility because of the 'tethered cord' in his spine, but at this point in his life, he can walk with callipers and walking sticks.

It's a good job that they can both walk, especially as we sample the Paris underground where passengers have to trek quite a long way to get to the platform. My feet are hurting and my arm is aching from dragging a small suitcase-on-wheels behind me, which contains all our bits and bobs for the overnight couchette.

The train glides into the bustling station and I have to take a second look.

It's a double-decker. I'd only ever seen a double-decker bus before. *Crikey, I didn't see that coming.*

As for young Tim, he's the model of good behaviour as we hike through the Paris underground, revelling in the experience of being in a different country, and a ride on a double-decker train.

As we wrap up our day, we visit the Eiffel Tower and gaze skywards at the awesome structure. Halfway up, enormous vibrant orange letters catch our attention, reminding us of the ticking countdown: only 211 days remain until the year 2000. Standing there, we can't help but feel a mix of anticipation and nostalgia as we witness this historic moment in time.

We queue up and ascend in the lift, but Don's vertigo overcomes him at the *premier étage* (first stage) of the Tower and his feet become like lumps of lead. He comes to a complete halt and can't walk any further, slumping down onto his knees to avoid being sick. He feels very queasy and cannot move. Mind you, he does treat me to a meal on the Tower though—a box of frites for 4 francs.

No one bats an eyelid at Don hunched down on all fours, so we leave him to rest while the three of us brave it up to the 2nd stage. It's a *long* way down as we peer through the viewing window, and I'm feeling somewhat funny in the tummy myself. Don wouldn't enjoy being up here. The people below look like ants.

We don't go up any higher and return to Don just as he is being escorted off the Tower by some helpful guards. He's feeling rather nauseous, but once he's back on the ground, he soon perks up.

A street artist accosts us into purchasing a cartoon drawing of young Tim for 5 francs. Tim is cock-a-hoop with it.

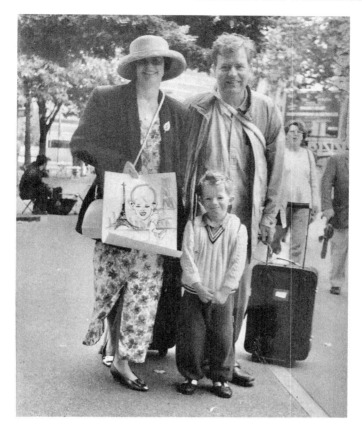

Despite Don's hiccup on the Tower, we sense that the day has gone well and we round it off by quaffing a refreshing drink back at La Bercy.

It's my 40th birthday. How grand to spend one's 40th birthday in Paris!

I indulge in a *Kir Royale* to celebrate, which costs 6 francs. I'd long wanted to try a *Kir Royale* (champagne and *Creme de Cassis*) after I'd learnt about the drink several years before when touring Belgium with the City of Birmingham Symphony Chorus. My singing companion would drink nothing else.

'*Kir Royale s'il vous plaît*,' she would order every time from the waiters as we bistro-crawled our way through Ghent.

'*Stella pour moi s'il vous plaît*,' was my regular tipple

according to my budget, so I never got to try her recommendation.

Now, as I finally get to taste this superb cocktail, I savour every bubbly mouthful.

Before boarding the train, we enjoy a meal in the Garden Restaurant at the station.

'*Bon appétit*,' the waiter utters rapidly as he places our meals before us. I just about recognise it as it comes out as "b'nappetty".

'What did he say?' enquires Don.

'He wishes us a good appetite.'

We then board the couchette train, and we are excited—next stop Fréjus!

But as we reach our cabin, we are in for a shock.

7. LA COUCHETTE

We are sharing a six-berth cabin with two strangers.

We are not expecting this at all, although it is standard practice in the 2nd class couchettes which Geoff has booked for us.

Inside the tiny compartment are six bunks, three on each side. Geoff and Don sleep on the bottom bunks. I sleep in the middle above Don, and Tim sleeps on the top bunk above me, which he thinks is great fun. The French couple sleep above Geoff with the man in the middle bunk and the woman on the top bunk.

I have a fitful night's sleep, as does Geoff. Don doesn't sleep at all. He worries about these two interlopers: who are they and can they be trusted? Will they steal from us while we are asleep?

Tim sleeps like a log.

Don needn't have worried at all, and his misgivings evaporate as we disembark from the train at 7 a.m. in Fréjus.

The morning sunlight gently bathes the surroundings, casting a warm glow on the honey-coloured villas that dot the landscape. Tall and slender poplar trees sway gracefully in the warm breeze. The statuesque palm trees add a touch of tropical grandeur to the scene and the shimmering sea, a pure azure blue, oozes the tranquillity of this coastal paradise.

Welcome to Provence! It's glorious. We are in love with the place already and into a continental breakfast at Fréjus station, by which time our Daewoo has been driven off the train and is ready and waiting for us. Off we go to our villa and revel in the resplendent coastal drive to Mandelieu La Napoule.

Geoff's daughter, Erica, meets us at Mandelieu in her white pickup truck and we follow her to the villa. Up, up, up we ascend the winding road, higher and higher, navigating each bend, our anticipation growing. Finally, we reached our destination—the villa. Instantly, I'm spellbound by its charm and the surrounding breathtaking vistas that stretch endlessly before us. It's magical.

Erica leaves us to unpack and settle in and announces she will join us later that evening with her partner Matt, who will cook us a barbecue. How kind.

Because I'm a nosey parker, I waste no time exploring this fascinating villa and I make a surprising discovery.

8. THE VILLA

The villa is built onto a rock face.

I'm surprised to find out that the rock forms the back wall of the utility room. I learn this by searching out where the washing machine is and I see the rock wall is oozing tiny rivulets of water. I'm shocked (thinking how awful it would be to discover water like that in my home), but Geoff assures me it's perfectly normal for this type of property.

The rest of the villa is fabulous. What can I say? As soon as I clap my eyes on it, I could live there in a heartbeat. It's a honey-coloured two-storey building with lavender-coloured shutters, situated high on a hill in a lane called *Les Terres du Soleil* (The Lands of the Sun) close to the delightful village of Capitou. I love it.

After unpacking, I put on a CD of Bach French Suites that I'd brought with me, pour a glass of wine that Erica kindly left in the fridge, and look out at the expansive scene from the window. At home in Brixham we also have a lovely sea view, but the view from the villa encompasses Cannes, several islands and an airstrip. We gaze, fascinated, watching the planes take off from Cannes Mandelieu Airport - especially Don, who, although he refuses to fly, is fascinated by the planes strutting their stuff.

Outside, the villa boasts a delightful patio adorned with an infinity pool alongside a bubbling jacuzzi, which entices us to sink into its warm embrace. It is exotic. We are enamoured by the infinity pool and as we swim through its waters, our eyes are transported not only across the shimmering ripples but far beyond into the distant panorama.

Despite Don's paralysis, he's able to wriggle along on his bottom into the pool every day without nosey onlookers (though this doesn't always put him off going into public pools or the sea).

However, our resident villa gecko that parks itself on the stair wall alarms Don and makes him somewhat unsure of it. But he soon accepts this intruder as part and parcel of French life in Provence (though no doubt the gecko sees *us* as the intruders).

The scene at night is also breathtaking, as the glimmering, shimmering lights of Cannes cast a magical glow upon the far-reaching panorama, resembling a whimsical wonderland. We witness a spectacular electric storm where jagged bolts of lightning slice through the sky, cutting it in two. The serene nights exude a gentle warmth, accompanied by a plethora of stars that adorn the heavens, while a resplendent, waning moon adds to the enchantment.

One night I show the bright crescent moon to four-year-old Tim through the window before putting him to bed.

'Look at the moon, it's so bright,' I coo.

'Oh,' he says in a sad little voice. 'It's broke.'

Well, I guess that's one way of describing a half-moon.

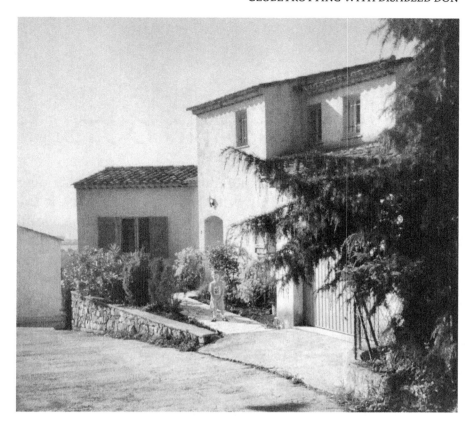

The villa

9. THE UP AND OUTS

During Geoff's many visits to France to see his daughter over the years, he had hooked up with a group of ex-pats at the Anglican Church in Cannes. On Sunday, the 13th of June, we all attend the church service there—though surely the main focus of attention is the sumptuous and scrumptious "bring and share" lunch afterwards, accompanied by copious amounts of wine. *Of course!*

It's a magnificent feast, the centrepiece being an enormous succulent whole salmon with all the trimmings, along with baguettes, exquisite cheeses, colourful salads and tasty *galettes.*

Everyone is super friendly and I get into conversation with an elegant lady called Virginia, who tells me about the work of the church and how it ministers to the "up and outs" in the local area.

'The up and outs?' I probe, interested in the incongruity.

'Yes, there are many up and outs in the French Riviera,' she advises. 'Very affluent people who are extremely sad, lonely and searching for true happiness and the meaning of life.'

'Oh. Hmm. Interesting. I guess money isn't everything.' *Surely being up and out in Provence is far better than being "Down and Out in Paris and London"? ...George Orwell, eat your heart out!*

Tim, dressed in one of his many stylish Verbaudet[1] outfits I'd purchased by mail order, looks very French. But Geoff disapproves of this attire. He considers it to be pretentious, and an unnecessary display of ostentatiousness. But I love it.

We enjoy several of these ex-pat gatherings, all ending in

lots of food and wine, and after one such boozy lunch at the home of Virginia for a "bible study", we move on for afternoon tea at the home of a lady called Philo who lives in a tiny townhouse in Biot. Afterwards, everyone visits the glassworks in Biot and watches them blowing glass.

Biot Glass is famous for deliberately capturing bubbles in the glass, which gives it a unique style. In the late 1950s, Éloi Monod, an engineer and ceramist, established the technique to trap bubbles intentionally in hand-blown glass. Normally the bubbles are a flaw, but Monod transformed them into a thing of beauty within the glass.

'We're off to Montecarlo tomorrow,' announces Geoff to the group before we all go our separate ways. 'We're taking the *Petit Train* around Monaco.'

'Good-oh,' says Virginia. 'That's the place where the residents ensure their lawns are mown to a specific height - not too short and not too long - but just right. *Parfait!*'

Seriously? We never got to see any residential lawns in Monaco, but judging by the size of the yachts in the harbour, I could well believe they made sure their grass was mown "not too short".

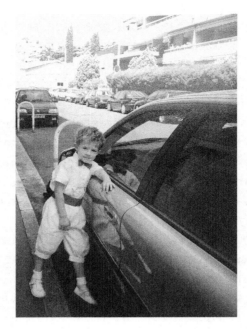

*Cool dude - Tim looking very dapper in his Verbaudet outfit,
cummerbund and all, leaning against the Volvo hire car
outside the Anglican Church in Cannes. (I parked the car
well, I thought - well done Reginald Molehusband[2]).*

[1] *Verbaudet is a French brand that offers an exclusive range of
clothing and accessories for children.*

[2] *Reginald Molehusband was a fictional character in a 1960s
public information film. He was depicted as the UK's worst driver
when he came to parallel parking his Austin 11 car.*

10. CAPITOU & A BOAT RIDE

Our days are very much governed by Geoff's disability in that he needs to lie down and have a snooze each day at 3 p.m. because he gets buzzing in his ears and starts feeling dizzy. But this routine works out well for all of us and we settle into a relaxed timetable enjoying leisurely morning coffee, followed by a pleasant lunch somewhere.

After lunch, a brief visit to either the beach at Cannes or La Napoule for an hour is in order before Geoff takes his nap. Even though he isn't a particularly beach-type person (walking on sand is difficult for both him and Don with their disabilities), he's considerate of young Tim and makes the effort to join us by the sea. We are impressed with the top-notch accessible parking on Cannes seafront, which helps us during our beach visits.

Late afternoons and evenings see us back at the villa in the pool and jacuzzi, relaxing with a glass of wine (or two). We go shopping one day while Geoff is taking his afternoon nap, but we discover that not only is Geoff taking his siesta, but the rest of Provence is too and all the shops are closed until 5 p.m. I am not well pleased.

Geoff had enthused about the village of Capitou, and we have to agree it is utterly delightful. We enjoy leisurely morning coffees there and watch the locals play the game of *Pétanque* (boules) in the square. This is a rare and special treat for our family, sampling French life.

In the quaint village, the *boulangerie* beckons with its aroma of freshly baked bread and tantalising sweet treats. The sight of intricate pastries and golden baguettes is enticing. Moreover, the *Fixe Prix* (fixed price) lunches, with their affordable and satisfying options, add another layer of culinary bliss. And let's not forget the Mandelieu market, where the aroma of succulent rotisserie chickens wafts through the bustling crowds, drawing me in. These simple pleasures bring us much joy.

On a couple of evenings, we dine out with Erica and Matt at the Marine Bar in Cannes (fondly known as "Schumacher's" by the locals because the owner looks like the German racing driver, Michael Schumacher) and the conversation turns to Erica and Matt's upcoming visit to Le Mans. Both she and Matt love car racing and they visit Le Mans every year. She also tells us we'll be having a barbecue on our last night up *Le Grand Duc.*

'Oooh, I'm excited,' announces Erica, sipping her Merlot.

'Me too, I love barbecues,' I respond.

Erica gives me a sideways glance.

'I mean about going to Le Mans,' she corrects.

Bump...of course, silly me! A barbecue up Le Grand Duc is no match for Le Mans!

The following day, Geoff insists we pay a visit to one of the enchanting Lerin islands. We eagerly board the ferry and make our way to Île Saint-Honorat, a haven where a close-knit community of Cistercian monks resides.

As soon as we set foot on the island, we're bathed in an acute sense of tranquillity. The sight of the breathtaking abbey against the backdrop of lush woodlands and serene beaches is nothing short of mesmerising.

The delicate aroma of blooming lavender, planted row upon row, envelops us, and the absence of traffic creates a harmony of calmness and quiet.

If I could relive one moment in Provence, it would undoubtedly be here, in this place of profound peace and natural splendour.

11. ALL GOOD THINGS...

Our time in the French Riviera is drawing to a close.

We spend a few more days swanning around Cannes and the beach at La Napoule and I cram in some last-minute shopping. As well as the smaller boutiques, I also love all the larger French outlets - *Decathlon, Carrefour,* and *E. Leclerc.* I stock up on *Crème de Cassis* and some bubbly, which is very cheap so that I can make *Kir Royales* at home, as well as a few bottles of Merlot at 2 francs a bottle - bargain!

I have a weakness for buying drinking vessels, whether they be glassware, pottery or china. The shapes and designs in the French outlets are exquisite and so cheap, and I buy many pieces.

We have no further accidents in the hire car and by the 18th of June, our repaired Daewoo is ready for us to collect from Sixt in St Raphael where we have to return the hire car. *It's time to face the consequences and admit to the damaged wing mirror.* I'm feeling nervous.

A smartly dressed assistant greets us and hands me the keys to our Daewoo. I show him the wing mirror - smashed and dislodged - explaining what had happened, but it was nothing to him.

'It is all covered in ze insurance, Madame,' he assures me. ''Ave no worries,' is the response I get over the shattered mirror.

Well, that was easy.

However, we've had a very accident-prone time at the villa. I've broken the handle off a lovely vintage teacup by placing it in the dishwasher incorrectly (well, in my defence, I'm not used to using a dishwasher, though I'm determined to get one of these amazing appliances for my kitchen when I get home - I love it), and Don has broken a vase and a beer glass. He's normally rather clumsy, often spilling and breaking things, and the words "I've had an accident" are one of his frequent mantras. Poor Erica will have to explain all that to the owners, and we give her some francs to pay for the damage along with our profuse apologies.

On our final evening, we join Erica and Matt, and some of their friends, for the barbecue at the *Le Grand Duc*. The setting lives up to its grand name, with breathtaking views and a vibrant atmosphere, making it the perfect ending to our vacation. As the evening unfolds, Erica and Matt craft a lavish feast fit for royalty, tantalising our senses. It rounds off with Erica's homemade cherry pie, which steals the spotlight. I've never eaten a cherry pie before, let alone tasted cherries so sweet yet tart at the same time—a scintillating fusion of flavours.

Thank you, Erica and Matt, for your kind hospitality.

It's time to head back home. We pack up with even more luggage piled up between me and Tim. We have a long drive ahead because we are not putting our car on the couchette train this time. It will take us four full days to get home.

We set off on the 20th of June, driving to the Hotel Campanile at Thiers. Geoff has not booked any accommodation on the way home because he is confident that we will get rooms, but this plan falls apart when we arrive at Chartres and discover that the Hotel Campanile there is full.

It's a further 24-mile drive to Dreux Campanile, where relief washes over us on discovering there are rooms available. We savour the last pickings of French culture and cuisine during the tail end of our vacation, and the next day we drive to the

Cherbourg Campanile via Caen, boarding the ferry at 8.45 a.m. to Poole on the 23rd of June.

What an adventure for us "staycationers"!

Unforgettable.

We are now full-blown Francophiles.

PART TWO - THE FRANCOPHILES RETURN

12. BON VOYAGE

When we arrive home, the weather is glorious.

'Why did we travel to the South of France when it's just as beautiful here?' observes Don as we sip our morning coffee on our patio, looking out across Torbay at the azure sea and sky, with Thatcher Rock glistening in the distance.

But there's no denying that we are infatuated with the South of France—we adore its differences, its culture, the food, and the ambience that engulfs us as we soak up the way of life there. As the winter months press in, a longing to return creeps up on us—plus the *Kir Royales* I try to make at home are rubbish compared to the ones in France.

We had casually dropped it to Geoff that we'd be happy to travel with him to Provence and stay in the villa any time. But no repeat offer is forthcoming from Geoff or his daughter. I guess it's no surprise: after nearly killing Geoff when I'd driven on the wrong side of the road, then putting him in mortal danger by travelling in a vehicle piled high with luggage, plus traumatising him when Don drove over *"une grande pierre,"* triggering his vulnerable emotions and then wrecking some of the crockery and glassware in the villa, they surely must feel we are unsuitable travel companions.

The winter passes, as does spring, and in June 2000 we stay with Geoff in Wimborne. Don has known Geoff for many years and we always spend a week or two at his bungalow every year, staying in the spare room.

While we are there, Don develops an infection in his left foot and he becomes extremely unwell as the infection spreads to his glands. This can sometimes happen in people with spina bifida. Don has no sensation in his feet and he cannot feel any pain. We go to A&E at Poole Hospital, and they admit Don straightaway and administer intravenous antibiotics. He spends a week there and has a marvellous room all to himself overlooking Poole Harbour.

Then Geoff comes to stay with us in Brixham for a week in August 2000 and announces that he's off to France for a month with one of his lady friends called Beth. Geoff has several of these female companions (all strictly platonic) - an entourage of mature ladies who have befriended him, taking him under their wing, and vice versa. He regularly entertains them all together for marvellous dinner parties at his modest home. Despite his disability after the stroke, Geoff is a remarkable cook and a whizz in the kitchen. His Sunday roasts are legendary, and his apricot crumbles are mouthwatering.

At the end of the week, over a sandwich lunch on our front patio, Geoff tells us Beth will drive from her home in Ringwood, Dorset to pick him up in Brixham and drive to Plymouth to get the car ferry to Roscoff. They'll be touring through France, staying in various *auberges* (inns).

And that's just how it happens: the indomitable Beth, *une femme formidable* if ever there was one, arrives in her bright red shiny convertible sports car with the top down and she and Geoff drive off into the sunset. Geoff's silk scarf blows in the wind like Isadora Duncan's, and with his right hand in the air waving us farewell, they disappear down the hill with a "toot toot" from the horn.

Bon voyage, Geoff and Beth.

We surely now know if we want to visit France once more, we will have to travel on our own, Geoff-less.

So Don sets about planning our next French holiday for 2001. We are in love with Mandelieu (fondly known as *Capitale du Mimosa)* and have decided to head there again. We so wanted to feast our eyes on the vibrant yellow blooms, but by the time we arrive in early summer, the floral feast will be over.

Don books a self-catering apartment on a large holiday

complex in Mandelieu for late May/early June for three whole weeks covering the half-term break. Tim has started school and we will now have to get special permission from his headteacher so that he can take time out and miss two weeks of his lessons. Financial penalties for parents taking their children off on holiday during school term time are looming, but we get away with it.

13. FRANCE 2001

In June 2001, with our Daewoo estate car packed up to the hilt, we set off once again to Provence, boarding the ferry in Plymouth which is just over an hour's drive away from our home in Brixham. We're always on a bit of a limited budget so this time we skip the overnight sleeper couchette from Paris to Fréjus, and will drive the 700-plus miles to Provence using various autoroutes through Nantes, Toulouse and Sète, staying at the affordable *Première Classe* hotels along the way. They're cheaper and more basic than the Hotel Campaniles we stayed at with Geoff, but there's no free villa waiting for us this time in Provence.

After arriving at Roscoff, we begin an uneventful journey down to Nantes, a massive city, which we drive through, stopping and starting our way through the busy road. I witness several large multi-storey buildings with people leaning out of the windows. Women in hijabs and young men holding toddlers, grabbing some fresh air, looking down at the traffic below. They spread their food supplies and drinks along the window ledges outside to keep cool in the evening shade.

We discover the amazing *Aires.* These are glorified service stations dotted throughout the journey where we can refresh. Mind you, my jaw dropped in disbelief as I encountered the unisex toilet, awkwardly hovering over a sink in the ground to relieve myself. I didn't like that at all.

Continuing our journey to Toulouse, we navigate the streets in search of the elusive N126, feeling a slight sense of disorientation. The city reveals a picturesque river, its waters glistening under the golden sunlight. The blooming flowers heighten the allure of the surroundings, but we choose to forge ahead, eager to reach our next destination.

After another exhausting day of driving, we arrive at the enchanting city of Sète. As we step out of the car, the gentle breeze carries the scent of the nearby sea. The picturesque canals, adorned with vibrant flowers and bustling with life, greet us with their charming appeal. The soft murmur of conversation and laughter wafts along the canal, as people enjoy their meals in the many alluring restaurants that line the streets.

Sète feels strangely familiar, reminiscent of our beloved fishing port, Brixham, albeit on a much grander scale. It even boasts a "high town" and a "low town" like Brixham, evoking a sense of nostalgia. In Brixham, the lower part around the harbour is affectionately known as "fish town", while the upper part nestled amongst the green hills is called "cow town." Don and Tim enjoy a bit of crabbing before we check into our *Première Classe* hotel, which isn't as classy as the Campaniles, but it's adequate.

On the following day, we head to the beach, but the gusty wind dominates the atmosphere, sending grains of sand flying in all directions and into every nook and cranny. The relentless wind howls in my ears, drowning out the soothing sound of the waves. Constant gusts irritate me, leaving me feeling restless and unable to fully enjoy the experience. Windy beaches just aren't my cup of tea.

We set off for Provence and I begin to catastrophise. I become anxious about the type of accommodation Don has booked in Mandelieu. Will the apartment be a tiny, shabby old thing, the French equivalent of an outdated, cheap Butlin's holiday camp?

14. THE APARTMENT

I needn't have worried. Our contemporary and roomy apartment is on a delightful holiday complex, nestled amidst a picturesque landscape enveloped by tranquil canals. This idyllic setting offers an ideal haven for Don and Tim to indulge in their fishing activities.

We check in and find our apartment. Before I can begin to relax and unwind, I always have a thing about unpacking everything. Don and Tim are excited and leave me to unpack while they head off for the pool. Even though Don can't walk without callipers and a walking stick, he can (at this point in his life) shuffle along on his bottom to the edge of the pool and slink in (mind you, getting back out is a bit of a different matter).

'I'll join you in a mo,' I say as they go off with the blow-up boat, paddle and blow-up beach ball while I put away all the food we'd stocked up on at *Carrefour* (my favourite French supermarket).

Finally, when I have everything in its place, I squeeze into my swimsuit, grab a towel and head off to join them.

But they're not in the pool, or around the pool.

Where on earth are they?

I'm hot, tired and long for a cooling swim, but am eager to find them in case they're wondering where I am. So off I go, mooching around the complex and discover there are two pools—a large one for adults, and a much smaller one for young children. I find the children's pool and sure enough, there they are, but what I'm not expecting is the sight that greets my eyes.

15. DON - THE KIDDULT

There, in the middle of the children's pool, is Don floating on Tim's tiny blow-up boat in six inches of water (I kid you not!)

'You're not supposed to be in *that* pool. It's for kids!' I chide.

'Nobody minds, darling. You worry too much. Come on in, it's lovely.'

Thankfully, there's no one else around to witness the embarrassing spectacle. *Good job we're here before the schools break up.* I swap Don with Tim before we head for the larger pool where I can have my long-awaited swim.

We are overjoyed with the site, and even though we missed the mimosa, the complex is bursting with vibrant, cerise-blooming bougainvillea. It is spectacular.

We are close to all our favourite places: Cannes, Capitou, and of course our beloved beach at La Napoule with its castle ruins. However, it has to be said that Don isn't at all sure about the French women sunbathing on the beach TOPLESS, achieving a nice even tan on their small, neat breasts. He thinks this display of nudity is dreadfully immodest. But he soon accepts this behaviour as the French way of life, and after a few days doesn't even notice them.

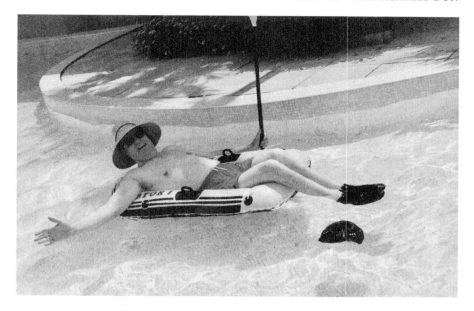

Don in the kiddies pool

16. NICE IS NOT NICE

'What are boysons?' Don asks me as we drive into Nice.

'Boysons?'

'Yes, up there on that kiosk,' he points to it as we drive past:

Boissons ~ Sandwiches ~ Frites

'That's pronounced bwahssohn! Not boysons. It means drinks. Your French is terrible. Didn't you ever learn it at school?'

'No?' he replies as a question as if he should have. He was born in 1945, and no one taught his generation French at all. Well, certainly not at state schools in inner city Birmingham where Don grew up. Even if he had, Don's education had been extremely patchy because of his many stays in hospital throughout his secondary school years.

Until he was 11 years old, Don's disability didn't affect him physically and he could run and jump like any other child. It was only as he grew taller throughout adolescence that his disability became worse. The spina bifida stretched the tendons in his legs and affected his walking as he grew into his 6' 2" adult height.

Bowel and bladder issues also kicked in as a teenager and frequent infections would cause many hospitalisations. At one point, the physicians suspected a tumour inside his lump, and Don had an experimental operation, cutting it open, but there was no tumour, and they couldn't do anything to untangle the cords. The operation put him in a wheelchair and it was months before he could walk again.

Don had to take his GCEs in hospital tutored by primary school teachers who had never taught to that level before, but they obtained the syllabuses and helped Don pass his exams.

I'm 14 years younger than Don, and I began learning French, aged 11, in the final year of primary school.

My school, St Lawrence Church of England Primary in Birmingham, had employed a mature French lady to visit us once a week and teach us elementary French. She was an exceedingly elegant woman with her stylish clothes and blond coiffed hair formed into an impeccable beehive bun. I wish I could remember her name.

Looking back, teaching 11-year-olds French was perhaps rather visionary of Birmingham Education Authority. Perhaps they'd foreseen closer ties with Europe, especially with decimalisation looming in 1971.

The first thing our French teacher taught us was our own name in French.

It got us all hooked.

It was personal now.

My name - Dawn - is *Aurore* in French.

I loved it.

Aurore. It sounded so...French.

'Je m'apelle Aurore,' I would mutter, *'Je m'apelle Aurore'.*

It was otherworldly.

I had a new identity.

Glamorous and different.

I was no longer a working-class kid from a council estate in Birmingham called Dawn Smith. I was *Aurore.* I was my name and my name was me - the early morning gleam, luscious and full of promise...*Oh well, dream on!*

But it was that simple thing that sparked my love of the French language, and in my teenage years, I studied it to 'O' Level standard at secondary modern school. Despite having no gift for speaking or understanding French due to my lack of linguistic aptitude, I found it a very musical language, and it sang to my heart.

But back to our holiday.

We hate Nice.

Our expectations of this place are completely misconstrued.

We envisioned something exotic.

A place of beauty.

Dreamy.

All the movie stars, the wealthy, and the famous flock to Nice for their vacations, don't they? It's surely a heavenly paradise, isn't it?

Yet, it's simply an energetic, overwhelming city with a sprawling six-lane motorway echoing alongside the glistening sea. The most delightful aspect is observing the roller skaters swiftly glide along the promenade, their efforts to stay fit palpable in the air.

Have I missed something about this place? I need a larger budget to visit the expensive boutiques and enjoy the wonderful shopping malls with posh overpriced shops, and we don't know the city at all, so after driving along the motorway on the seafront we pull over and look for somewhere else to explore nearby instead.

Maybe it's us? Perhaps we're too old for *Nice*, and six-year-old Tim is too young? It just isn't the place for us as a family, and we cannot connect with it.

We redeem the day somewhat when we discover that there's an art gallery not far away—the *Musée National Message Biblique Marc Chagall*. We both like art and think that Tim's school would approve if he could write a bit in his diary about such an educational visit.

Marc Chagall was a Russian Jew (his real name was Moishe Shagal). He once said of his childhood that "Lines, angles, triangles, squares, carried me far away to enchanting horizons," and certainly as an artist in Paris, he used those lines and angles imaginatively to evoke Russian village life in his fantastic creations.

His artistic influence was cubism. We find his artwork to be wonderfully unique, to say the least.

And colourful.

It was an interesting end after a disappointing start to the day. *Thank you, Monsieur Chagall.*

17. ITALIE

'What does inter-dit mean?' Don enquires (pronouncing *"interdit"* phonetically as "inter" and "dit").

We are driving along the E80 autoroute from La Napoule on our way to Italy, and overhead is a sign announcing *"Italie Interdit"*.

'I don't know. I haven't come across that word before. I think it's pronounced *anterdee*.'

'Well, it's no use knowing how it's pronounced if you don't know what it means,' observes Don.

Touché.

'Drat, I've left our pocketbook of French phrases back at the apartment,' I discover as I rummage through the glove compartment and my handbag. 'I know the word *dit* is a French verb meaning "said", and as for "inter", well that must mean the same as in English, like interrupt, or interchangeable...but inter-said? Nope, doesn't make sense. I don't know what it means.'

'Well, we'll keep going,' announces Don, ever-optimistic. 'Can't be anything too bad. Everyone else is going the same way.'

It's the 4th of June—my birthday again. What a good excuse to visit San Remo in Italy, just a mere hour and a half away from La Napoule. Spending my birthday abroad is becoming a pleasant habit and we're looking forward to sampling some Italian life—*pizza, vino, gelato* and an enjoyable time on the beach at San Remo.

The E80 autoroute goes to Italy through Nice, Monaco, and Menton, then on past the Italian border to Ventimiglia, and

San Remo. We drive through a seemingly endless tunnel, carved into the heart of a colossal mountain. *It must have taken a whole load of explosives to blow through this.*

As we emerge on the other side, we find ourselves travelling across a remarkably high viaduct and Don's vertigo overcomes him. He slows right down to 15km per hour as he grips the steering wheel.

'You've got to try and go faster than this!' I encourage him, looking behind us as car horns begin blaring.

'I can't! I keep thinking I'm going to drive over the edge…I feel sick.'

'Just keep calm and keep driving,' I coo. 'Take some deep breaths.'

The French drivers are not happy one bit, and headlights start flashing, accompanying their beeping horns.

We make it over the viaduct at a snail's pace and out onto firm terrain where Don soon perks up and we pick up some speed.

We travel over several of these lofty viaducts, all with the same result along with frequent signs announcing "*Italie Interdit*".

'It must mean something isn't right. Look! There's a red cross over the lane to Italy. I think it means it's not possible to get there. Maybe we shouldn't go to Italy today. What do you think?' I observe as the traffic becomes sparse.

We keep going towards Italy.

This is a big mistake. We end up on a tiny coastal road because the autoroute to Italy is blocked off from the autostrada at the A10.

'Do you think we should go back, darling?' I murmur.

'We've come this far, we may as well get to San Remo now'.

Undaunted and determined to spend my birthday in Italy, we continue on a slower coastal road through Ventimiglia. All the time, Tim has been golden in the back seat, amusing himself and enjoying the mild drama of the tooting horns.

We arrive in San Remo mid-afternoon, a tad exhausted and

frustrated. There's just enough time to enjoy a *gelato* and a happy hour or two on the beach. I unload our deck chairs and beach stuff. But out of nowhere, a young, tanned man with curly black locks flowing in the sea breeze is striding towards me, waving his arms.

18. NO! NO! NO! SAN REMO

'No! No! No!' he shouts at me. It appears *"no"* in Italian is the same as it is in English, so there's no misunderstanding there. It turns out the beach is *privato* (private), and members of the public are not welcome there. Don tries to explain we've come a long way and just want an hour on the beach, but language is a problem and the beach attendant is having none of it. So I have to put everything away again. Don submits to this blow. Normally he would be quite jaunty and challenge it in his jocular manner, especially as the private beach is empty with no one on it, but he's been subdued by his vertigo over the viaducts, and he's not in the mood to haggle with belligerent beach attendants.

'No! No! No!' This time a car park attendant comes up to us and points out we can't park in the beach car park either, so we have to move onto the road. By now we are hot, hungry and thirsty. Determined to salvage something of the day, I wander off to check out the food outlets along the seafront. An authentic Italian takeaway pizza washed down with an ice-cold lager would help to ease the disappointment. But I'm in for a surprise which catches me completely off guard.

19. EUROPEAN DISUNION

All the prices are in lira.

Stupid me! We have no lira.

I walk into a takeaway and show my French francs.

'No! No! No! Lira!' is the response from the cashier.

I go back to Don.

'I don't believe it. We should have got some lira! They don't take francs in Italy. Now what are we going to do?' I bemoan, feeling grumpy. 'We need to find a bank and draw some out with our credit card.'

'Surely that ice cream kiosk over there will take some francs? We're right on the border here.'

I saunter over, but all the prices are in lira.

'Francs?' I ask, hopefully, waving a five franc note.

'No! No! No!' says the server, shaking his head. *'Lira, per favore!'*

I go back to Don, 'Nope. We can't even buy a blummin' ice cream!'

Crikey, what a disaster.

I attempt to find a bank, but the language barrier asking for directions is too complicated and I give up.

By now, we just want to get back to our apartment. We're too frazzled to go hunting for a cash point. Poor little Tim is still an angel, and he thinks it's all a bit of an adventure—a sort of farce, witnessing his clueless parents who are traveller buffoons and utterly inadequate in a foreign country. Our visit to San Remo is a complete washout and we leave without enjoying any of its beauty.

Don drives back to our apartment on the coastal road as he can't face driving over the high viaducts again, and as soon as we cross the border, we find a place to eat at Mirazur—a brief respite from our disappointment.

Back on the road again after our meal, my bladder doesn't have far to go until it needs relief, so we stop off at Menton to find a loo. We park up on the seafront and I ask several people *"toilette s'il vous plaît?"* but they silently ignore me as if I don't exist. They are uncooperative and will not assist me in locating a public toilet at all. *How rude.* Or maybe the place is too posh to have such a thing as a public toilet? I have a very uncomfortable ride back to Mandelieu.

It's been an unsuccessful and wasted day. When I get back to the apartment, I find my phrase book and look up the word *interdit.*

It means "forbidden". Hey ho, there you go! It certainly brought an essence of *"Je ne sais quoi"* to my birthday in France that year (in the "indescribable" sense!)

20. AU REVOIR.....

The rest of our holiday passes smoothly. We make friends with the guests in the apartment next door to ours, a friendly German couple called Michael and Anna. We enjoy a barbecue with them and share some very pleasant *soirées* over coffee and wine, chatting late into the balmy evenings.

After a few glasses of wine that liberates their emotions, they shock us by disclosing that they feel shame about being German because of the Nazi history associated with their country and nationality. We tell them we have never even thought about such a thing and assure them they are not responsible for what happened in the Second World War. They are our friends.

We return to the captivating island of St. Honorat. Our previous visit with Geoff still lingers in our memory, beckoning us irresistibly, like a magnetic force. I tell Tim there will be monks on the island and after visiting the tranquil abbey, we walk the circumference of the island, culminating in a picturesque picnic at one of the bijou beaches.

'Where are the monkeys?' asks Tim.

'It's *monks*, Tim. The word is monks, not monkeys. We saw some of them in the abbey dressed in their robes,' I explain.

He's a tad disappointed, however, just like he was when we visited the Peak District in Derby once. 'Where are the pigs?' Tim had asked. 'It's peaks Tim, *peaks.* Not pigs.'

I love how children misinterpret adult words.

We conclude our holiday exploring the picturesque coastal path to Theoule-sur-Mer, where the salty breeze caresses the face, along with the scent of the sea. The vibrant colours of the Mediterranean landscape unfold beside the azure waters, blending seamlessly with the cerulean sky.

At a quaint seaside restaurant, I eagerly indulge in a steaming bowl of bouillabaisse. It's the best soup I've ever eaten in all my born days. The flavours are exquisite—it's an embodiment of culinary perfection and lingers in my memory.

Upon my father's recommendation, we explore Villefranche-sur-Mer. Having been entranced by its breathtaking landscape during his naval service in 1950, he insisted we witness its beauty firsthand.

Perched in the hills, reminiscent of Brixham, this town gradually ascends building by building above sea level, merging with the landscape. The honey-coloured dwellings, adorned with towering trees, create a dreamlike ambience. The exquisite chapels and churches add a touch of serenity to the already mesmerising surroundings. Regrettably, our time was limited, and we yearn for more moments to absorb this haven. Oh, what a magnificent port it would be to call home.

We revisit Cannes and embark on a delightful journey aboard Le Petit Train du Suquet, luxuriating in the breathtaking panorama of the town from an elevated vantage point. As the train ascends, we are greeted with awe-inspiring vistas, the sight of vibrant rooftops and charming streets stretching out before us. The rhythmic ding ding ding of the *petit train* bell harmonises with our excitement, creating a consonance of anticipation and pleasure. Reaching the top, we marvel at the grandeur of Cannes from this remarkable height.

These simple things might seem somewhat mundane to other travellers who've seen the sights of more exotic places, but to us, Provence is a fresh experience and a different culture. We love it all.

Apart from the fiasco in San Remo, our visit this time went smoothly, as did our journey home. And there were no disasters driving over large stones up the Alps this time. *Good-oh!* (as my father would have said). We had a merry time.

◆ ◆ ◆

A few months later, Geoff rings us up and he's in floods of tears again.

'The towers, the towers…' he sobs, his voice trailing off.

It is September 11th.

The scenes on our television of the Twin Towers falling touch us all and we will forever remember the year 2001 for reasons other than our French holiday #2.

21. A DAY TRIP TO FRANCE - 2002

'You'd love France, Dad,' Don says to his father. 'Would you like to come with us on a day trip?'

'Yes son, that'd be lovely,' he said, full of hope and expectation.

Don's father, Harold, is a widower and has never been abroad at all. So at the grand age of 89, Harold gets a passport and makes his very first trip to Europe.

We set off early from Brixham on a late summer morning along the A38 to Plymouth, sunshine all the way, and board the car ferry over to Roscoff. We're looking forward to spending time in France again, and I have my heart set on visiting *Carrefour* and *E. Leclerc,* then quaff a *Kir Royale* or two, and savour French fayre and food in a nice little French Bistro somewhere.

But from the start, Harold is not happy. I guess he's too old to change the habits of a lifetime. He likes what he likes, and he isn't interested in trying out new things in a foreign country.

From the time we park our car on the ferry and navigate our way up to the restaurant, things aren't to his taste at all. And sod's law, he *would* pick up a newspaper that's in French from the onboard shop, which doesn't help.

'Can't understand a bloody word of this!' he laments.

I buy him an English newspaper which keeps him happy for a couple of hours. For me, the holiday starts on the Brittany Ferry. They have a markedly French flavour with French things to buy along with some duty-free goodies. But Harold soon gets bored and misses his favourite soap opera *Neighbours*.

At Roscoff, he doesn't like any of the eating places or the food. There's no brown sauce for a start. Don gets out his map of France.

'I think we'll head to Morlakes,' says Don with confidence. 'It's bigger than Roscoff and there should be more choice of eating places,' he observes.

'Morlakes?' I double-check him.

'Yes Morlakes,' repeats Don, 'it's only about half an hour away.'

Morlakes?

Hmm, OK.

We set off again, hopeful that Morlakes would hold some good things for Harold.

After about ten minutes, I see a road sign to "Morlaix" and the penny drops.

'That's pronounced *morlay*,' I correct Don, 'not morlakes. Your French is terrible.'

Without incident, we arrive in Morlaix, a picturesque town built on three hills with quaint cobblestone streets. Seven-year-old Tim, good as gold as always, gets his micro-scooter out of the boot. He'll have fun riding that over the cobblestones. We all stretch our legs, and Don and Harold use two walking sticks each for extra safety.

As we amble through the charming alleys adorned with blossom, the tantalising aroma of freshly baked pastries wafts from the local patisseries. The sound of laughter and chatter echoes from the bustling bars and cafes that line the lively main square. However, despite the vibrant atmosphere, Harold is unmoved, finding no delight in the drinks served at the bars, leaving him thoroughly unimpressed. Half a mild is his favourite tipple, and he doesn't drink wine. Lager is not his thing. A pot of tea and a teacake is impossible to find, and we can't find a fish and chip shop anywhere. He is not a happy bunny.

To top it all, we have to suffer an overnight crossing back to Plymouth and sod's law would have it we're given sleeping bunks right next to the blasted engines. They keep us awake all night with the thud thud thud constantly thrumming away.

'Don't ever take me there again, son,' laments Harold. 'It's a bloody awful place,' is his verdict on France.

I shake my head in disbelief. *Well, you can't teach an old dog new tricks, as they say.*

Our trip to France with Harold is a complete flop.

As we drive off the ferry in Plymouth, we try to make it up to Harold and head for a fish and chip restaurant. We find one close to the Barbican - cod and chips all served up with mushy peas, white sliced bread and butter, with a big mug of steaming tea. It's right up Harold's street.

'Ooooh lovely, this is my kind of food,' says Harold as he picks up the sugar shaker, thinking it's salt and sprinkles it all over his chips...*oops.*

22. FRANCE & THE ALPS 2003

As the months wear on, our yearning for all things French (especially all things Provence) grips us once more. There's still no offer from Geoff or his daughter to stay in the villa. So we decide to go on our own again, Geoff-less (and, needless to say, Harold-less). We plan to travel during our favourite time of year - early summer at the beginning of June. We're able to get time off school for Tim once again, avoiding a fine on one condition: that Tim would write up a daily diary.

We set sail from Plymouth to Roscoff and use the toll-free roads over the Alps to avoid paying charges as we drive down the eastern side of France via Reims to Annecy, exploring the Alps before going on to Mandelieu La Napoule. Don has booked even cheaper accommodation at the budget "Formula 1" hotels (*hotelF1*) along the way.

The drive through France using the toll-free roads offers a diverse landscape. Initially, we navigate through a flat terrain adorned with charming towns peppered with traffic lights. As we progress southward, the scenery becomes more awe-inspiring with the emergence of majestic mountains and valleys which resemble a giant's tooth cavity. The drive is interminable, stretching endlessly before us.

It goes on and on along with the inevitable and many "Are we there yet?" questions from eight-year-old Tim. Don and I share the driving this time, and long-distance travelling by car is not one of my favourite pastimes. The drive is laborious, and I dislike it.

'If we ever come again, I'm not doing this higgledy-piggledy driving through all these towns and narrow mountain roads. It's much better to save up and pay for the autoroutes,' was my verdict as we finally pulled into Annecy after a seven-hour drive that day.

23. ANNECY

Our exploration of the Alps and Lac Leman make the long drive all worth it, with the exquisite Old Town of Annecy being our first stop. We are staying at the *Formula 1* hotel for several nights in the Haute-Savoie area. These basic hotels are more like hostels and it reminds me of holidays in the 1960s as I traipse off to the shower room with my wash bag and towel. The shower rooms are so tiny there's no way Don can use the facilities for showering, so it's a wash-down for him in our cramped bedroom.

By now, Don and Tim are well into fishing as a hobby and they're able to enjoy keeping "tight lines" at a French canal near the pretty town of Annecy, which has a maze of canals passing through it, giving it the charming name of the "Venice of the Alps".

All due credit to Don, he's done some research on the Alps. He discovers that the town of Annecy is near Lake Annecy, which is the second-largest lake in France. The shimmering, transparent waters of the lake invite us to take a refreshing swim, but the chilly temperature deters us, preferring to stroll along the promenade, accompanied by the rhythmic whir of Tim's micro-scooter.

It's the simple things that make the trip so pleasant, including a motorboat ride on the lake, and enjoying lunch in one of the many restaurants there.

We discover the delightful Sunday market in Annecy with bargains galore on the colourful stalls along the Old Town's streets and canals. It must be the most picturesque market on earth. France has just transitioned to using the *euro* and I get a lot more for my money with £1 equaling nearly 2 *euros.* I'm in shopping heaven.

Plus, being a *Carrefour* fan, I'm fascinated to learn that the *Carrefour* store - one of the biggest hypermarket chains in the world - first opened its doors in Annecy on January 1st, 1958 on the ground floor of a building named *"carrefour"*, which means "crossroads".

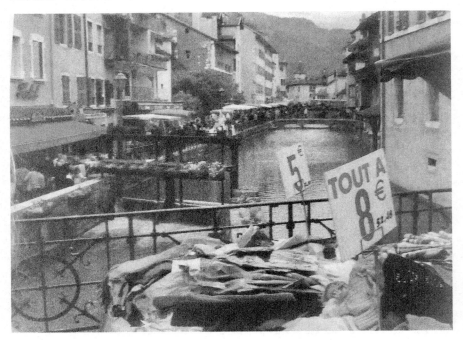

Sunday market in Annecy Old Town

24. LAC LEMAN (LAKE GENEVA)

From our base in Annecy, we take time to explore the towns around the Lac Leman (or Lake Geneva, as it's more commonly known) crossing the border to Vevey in Switzerland.

Then we time-travelled backwards to the 14th century with a visit to the delightful village of Yvoire. Don has to use two walking sticks here due to the many steps as we explore this exceptionally pretty place with its well-preserved medieval buildings, as well as its charming harbour. We could see why it has earned the name "gem of the lake."

Nestled within the village lies the enchanting *"Jardin des Cinq Sens"* (Garden of Five Senses), a captivating haven that beckons to awaken all the senses.

For the eyes, a kaleidoscope of colour.

For the nose, a delicate symphony of floral fragrances.

For the tongue, tiny fruits reminiscent of childhood.

For the ears, the whisper of water and sweet birdsong.

And for the touch, the soft and gentle lamb's ear.

A sensory experience to remember.

Regrettably, we missed out on this extraordinary garden, discovering its existence only after our departure. *Typical!*

A visit to Evian les Bains is on our planned itinerary. Located on the shores of Lake Geneva, it's a Spa town that has a history of being popular with royalty, including Edward VII and King Farouk of Egypt. And of course, it's famous for its mineral water. Evian is the brand name of bottled water familiar to many, and also one of my favourite face sprays to use during hot weather. But yet again, our incompetence as travellers lets us down and leads us into a spot of bother. We haven't done our homework…

25. G8

'Are those police?' I ask, taking off my sunglasses as if doing that will make them disappear.

'Yes, they're flagging us down.'

We stop.

The police don't speak good English, and I don't speak good French,

'Zhé huit sécurité,' is about all they can say, but we get the drift: there's an international conference taking place in Evian les Bains. We'd heard about the G8 summit from previous years where world leaders from eight countries come together to talk about global stuff - big names such as Jacques Chirac, Silvio Berlusconi, Vladimir Putin, Gerhard Schröder, Tony Blair and Dubya (aka George W. Bush). To think that these bigwigs were just a stone's throw away, probably enjoying a slap-up meal with caviar and canapés and quaffing top-notch champers in a posh hotel.

In 2001, just two years previously, the G8 summit had unfolded in Genoa, Italy. We'd read about it in the papers: the air was thick with tension as anti-globalist protestors flooded the streets, their voices echoing through the city. The atmosphere reeked of discontent and dissent. The scene was palpable with intense emotions, as the demonstrators made their presence felt, turning the event into a focal point of unrest. One protestor, Carlo Guiliano, was shot dead by a policeman.

So now, the police are keen to scrutinise all visitors to the town and make sure we aren't rebels. We convince them we're just holidaymakers, and the *gendarmes* decide that Tim, who's sitting in the back seat, isn't a subterfuge. They accept we are genuine tourists and not planning to blow up Evian les Bains, or protest and cause any trouble. They let us through.

At Evian, we are dazzled by the breathtaking high-powered fountains, as Tim stands amidst towering jets erupting from the ground. He thinks it is marvellous fun, and he's as high as a kite zigzagging through the water spouts. However, beyond that, we conclude that it's not a destination we would revisit. As inexperienced travellers, we lack the skill to fully engage in the art of sightseeing. Plus, compounded by the constraints of our budget, our ability to truly enjoy and savour new places becomes limited.

We conclude that visiting a mountain might hold more scenic interest for us...

26. MONT BLANC

So, before setting off south to Provence, we can't resist a visit to Chamonix and Mont Blanc (meaning "white mountain"). The area is so close it's a pity to pass it by, so we stop off for a picnic breakfast, parking up with a spectacular view.

Mont Blanc is the highest mountain in Europe and is the 11th tallest peak in the world. Each year between 20,000 and 30,000 climbers attempt to summit Mont Blanc, and yet it's one of the most fatal mountains on the planet. It's commonly known as the Death Mountain or the White Killer. Some estimates suggest it claims the lives of 30 people per year on average.

We board the *Le Train du Montenvers*, a delightful little red locomotive, and embark on a scenic journey up the mountain. As the train chugs along, the sights unfolding before our eyes are vast. The majestic and renowned *Mer de Glace* (Sea of Ice), France's largest glacier stretching 7km in length, comes into view. However, to my astonishment, the glacial expanse appears grey and tarnished, lacking the anticipated radiance. I had envisioned a glistening, ethereal sea of ice, adorned in pristine shades of white and bathed in luminosity. *What a disappointment.*

We then go into the glacier, walking right inside its gaping mouth, where it is dark, cool and a tad creepy. I was the only tourist wearing shorts and flip-flops.

27. LA NAPOULE

We head south to continue our holiday with a relaxing week at our favourite beach in La Napoule. Don was very proud to have found a good deal at a hotel right on the seafront.

The beach at La Napoule is a dream for us; the stretch of soft golden sand is complemented by the wonderfully warm, shimmering azure sea.

Next to the beach is the *Château de la Napoule*, a meticulously restored French castle where we can engross ourselves in the rich tapestry of its history and enjoy the gorgeous gardens—a veritable feast for the senses. Wandering through the enchanting grounds, we're besotted by the sights of vibrant flowers in bloom, the sound of birdsong reverberating all around, and the fragrant scent of nature's perfume mingling with the gentle sea breeze. We step into the cinematic world where the castle features as one of the main locations in the 1999 action movie *Simon Sez.*

Moreover, the proximity of La Napoule to all the amenities makes this corner of Provence even more enticing.

Parfait!

The main attraction, however, is by far the beach. The sea is at a temperature which Don can tolerate. Because of his health condition, cold water makes him feel jittery and strange, triggering his disability issues. And what a treat for us that the hotel is so close to the seafront. Everything is perfect in La Napoule, right?

28. THAT CERTAIN JE NE SAIS QUOI

'Did you tell them you're disabled?' I ask Don as I help him navigate the steps down into the strange room at the hotel. *The last thing we need is an accident or broken bones.*

'Yes, I rang the owner, but he didn't speak good English. I thought I'd made it clear.'

The hotel is quaint but not what we were expecting at all. This is a huge disappointment. Our room is most peculiar, and it's immediately obvious why we'd got it so cheap. It's higgledy-piggledy and dips down a few steps into a kind of semi-basement area with a strange, tiny ensuite bathroom which you have to climb up a few steps into. It's completely unsuitable for a disabled person with mobility issues, but we gave the owner the benefit of the doubt that he'd not understood Don's needs.

A decent room would have lifted the whole holiday. But it seems to be some kind of spare room they've put us in which is sunk into the floor, and even though it has an ensuite bathroom, it's all a bit of a squash and somewhat shabby-chic (more shabby than chic, though). Then, on top of that, to save some money, Don has booked us in for the room only, so that means we'll be scurrying around for a *boulangerie* and *fixe prix* (fixed price) lunches. And to rub salt into that wound, we have to pass all the other hotel guests enjoying their delicious French repasts in the hotel while we have to go out and find our meals. *Never mind, we can still enjoy this.*

One good thing, at least, is that it's close to the beach and, of course, Tim loves it. But Don is *not* a minimalist. As is typical for him, he has to have at least three of everything and a wide range, to boot, and the number of beach toys and accoutrements he has packed is no exception. He'd bought the lot: beach ball, loungers, blow-up boat, blow-up swimming ring, pump, beach games, fishing nets, snorkels and other beach gear. He is determined to have an absolute beach fest.

I'd been looking forward to some relaxing mornings or afternoons on the beach, sunbathing and reading, but it was not to be. I take 45 minutes and many trips to and from the car parked right on the seafront to carry all the beach gear down to the beach.

By the time I bring the last of the beach kit, Don is blowing up the boat with the pump and Tim is building sandcastles. I flop onto my lounger, sweating profusely.

At last. Time to relax and read my book.

'I'm a bit sinking, darling, I could do with a bite to eat,' announces Don, (the word 'sinking' being a Don-ism for 'I'm hungry').

Stone the crows! I can't sit down for five minutes!

'But I've only just sat down! I'll go in a mo,' I moan, picking up my book. But I can't relax, and conscious of my own hunger pangs, after five minutes I go off to buy baguettes, fillings, frites and drinks.

Back at the beach, I assemble a picnic lunch. On my last mouthful, Tim and Don decide they've had enough of the beach. So then I have to take all the beach gear back to the car bit by bit—another 45-minute job.

'*Sacré bleu!*' I curse, French style, as a tanty comes on. 'Why did you bring all this blasted beach gear? Everyone else just has a towel, a bucket and a spade. I can't unpack all this lot every time we come to the beach. I haven't even had time for a swim!' I whine as I help Don back to the sidewalk. His callipers and walking stick are of little use as he stumbles his way through the soft, silky sand.

It is no mean feat getting him back onto firm ground as

he hangs on to my right shoulder with one hand and uses a walking stick with the other. I could see why his peers at school had called him "rubber legs".

The numerous journeys to and from the beach made me forget to put any sun protection on my bare legs, which are now burnt. I spend a painful night smothered in Sudocrem.

29. RENDEZVOUS

I appreciate Don's effort to make the holiday an enjoyable experience for Tim with all the beach gear, but I'm glad to do something different the next day. We are still in touch with Erica and Matt, and they kindly invite us to their home near Mandelieu.

They live in a cave which is on the land of a villa that used to be a restaurant. It belongs to one of their clients who employs them to look after the property and grounds. Built into the rock face, Erica and Matt have kitted out the cave with a small lounge, a bathroom, a kitchen and one bedroom.

We settle down with a drink in their cosy lounge and watch the film *Ice Age,* which delights young Tim immensely. Indeed, it delights us all because Erica and Matt have one of the latest complete home movie set-ups and their enormous TV screen fills the entire wall of the cave, complete with the new-fangled "surround sound" speakers. It's like being in a real cinema and the sound effects are stupendous.

'This home movie gear is our main pleasure,' explains Erica. 'We don't spend on other luxuries, but we enjoy watching films on our big screen with surround sound.'

Fair enough.

We revel in the film and we all fall in love with Sid the Sloth and Scrat the Rat. Classic.

We then enjoy a meal out on their small patio, and Erica tells us that one of the boats she looks after could do with a run to keep the engine in good condition. She invites us to go on a boat ride around the Lérins Islands. What a treat.

Now, it might be that a boat ride around the Lérins Islands

is unremarkable to some travellers, but to us, it's a unique experience and we love it. Tim is tickled pink as he takes a turn at the wheel.

The shiny boat is swift as it bobs over the slightly choppy waves being churned up by a warm breeze. The sea reflects the azure sky, giving us the feeling of zipping through a blue sheet, occasionally interrupted by the distant view of the coasts. It is one of the highlights of our holiday.

On our way home, we embrace the enchanting atmosphere of Marine World in Antibes. The captivated audience gasps in awe at the antics and graceful spectacle of the acrobatic dolphins jumping and performing tricks.

As the sun begins to set, we continue our journey northwest through the alluring city of Carcassone. The majestic walls, adorned with over 50 towers, cast long shadows in the evening twilight. A symphony of laughter and joyful music surrounds us as we approach a mesmerising carousel, its colourful lights illuminating the night sky.

We return home without incident, and Tim's teacher expresses great admiration for the diary he has written, but the school explicitly states that trips abroad during term time are strictly prohibited.

With Don's no-fly status, we need at least three weeks for a trip to Provence. We do not want to go there in July and August, so it's curtains for holidays there for us during early summer.

PART THREE - MEMORIES OF THE ALHAMBRA

30. GLOBETROTTING WITHOUT DON

What does someone in a wheelchair do if they need the loo?

How do they board a plane?

How do they cross the road if the kerb is so high they can't get down it?

Can you board a coach if you're in a wheelchair?

Can you get into all the shops and cafes?

Are the doors wide enough?

Can you get onto all the buses and trains?

Can you get into a taxi?

As a non-disabled person, such questions weren't on my radar at all before I met Don.

Thankfully, accessibility is so much better than it used to be in many parts of the world. But things have not always been easy for disabled people, including the UK.

In the early 1990s, two disability activists - Barbara Lisicki and Alan Holdsworth - became trailblazers for disability rights in Britain, bringing about the Disability Discrimination Act of 1995 (now the Equality Act 2010).

During the early 90s, disabled individuals in Britain encountered numerous obstacles in various aspects of their lives. They faced difficulties in finding employment, accessing suitable housing, using public transport, and entering public buildings such as shops, restaurants, and cinemas.

At that time, it was commonly believed that disabled people should be the passive recipients of charitable donations. They were not seen as equal, independent citizens with legal rights.

But things began to change when disabled individuals flooded the streets, unleashing chaos with their impassioned protests: fastening themselves to public transport with chains, and wheelchair users barricading roads, their chants echoing loudly through the air.

The film *When Barbara Met Alan* depicts how the pungent scent of determination hung in the atmosphere as the protestors caused havoc, with police officers lifting disabled demonstrators from their wheelchairs and laying them on the ground. Amidst it all, the resounding cries for civil rights reverberated, highlighting the injustices they confronted. These protests ignited a fire within disabled individuals, revealing their newfound ability to wield influence upon lawmakers.

And it worked.

By the early 2000s, as Don began using a wheelchair more and more, accessibility was improving year after year, and when we began travelling abroad together, disabled people could access many more places.

Before I met Don, I hadn't travelled much at all and accessibility wasn't an issue that crossed my mind, nor had it been something my family had ever had to cope with.

My parents never went abroad as it was something that lower working-class families in the 1960s generally didn't do, mainly because it was too expensive, but also because culturally it wasn't the done thing. The Isle of Wight was the furthest we ever got across the sea.

There was one exception, though, and that was when I accompanied my father to Belgium in August 1972. I was 13 at the time, and we travelled by train from Birmingham to get the ferry from Dover to Ostend, and then onward by train to Mons. The reason for this adventure was that my cousin Ronnie (who was much older than me) was in the Royal Navy and based at S.H.A.P.E. (Supreme Headquarters Allied Powers Europe). He invited my father to visit him there, and it was decided I would go too while my mother and sister remained at home.

My father and I stayed with my cousin Ronnie, his wife and two daughters in their lovely, spacious flat on the S.H.A.P.E. complex in the picturesque village of Casteau, near Mons in Belgium.

My father, a passionate history lover, eagerly arranged a visit to *Breendonk* in Antwerp. This place, once a detention centre used by the Nazis during World War II, left an indelible mark on my memory. As we stepped inside, the grim sight of the dismal dormitories was stark. A heavy mix of mustiness and despair lingered all around. The visit opened my eyes to a harsh new reality.

On a more pleasant note, I soaked up the essence of the Continent awakening my awareness as I discovered the subtle nuances of their customs—from the way they presented a glass of tomato juice to the elegant ambience that surrounded it. In the UK, tomato juice is served simply, perhaps with a hint of Worcester sauce upon request.

However, in Belgium, the waiter delivered it in a tall, exquisite glass adorned with a delicate paper doyley beneath. A slice of lemon perched gracefully on the side, accompanied by delectable seasonings and a dainty stirrer. It was a small yet profound distinction, and I relished every sip. But we never went again and our next family holiday was in Weston-Super-Mare. It simply couldn't compare.

It would be 15 years later when my next trip abroad presented itself.

31. ACROSS THE POND

I joined the City of Birmingham Symphony Orchestra (CBSO) Chorus as a 2nd soprano in 1981. After leaving school, I studied music for three years with the hope of becoming a professional musician. However, things didn't go as planned, and I ended up working as a civil servant from nine to five instead.

Being part of the CBSO Chorus was a musical lifeline for me. It allowed me to perform music at a professional level, even though I was just an amateur chorister. Moreover, being a member of such a prestigious choir took me to parts of the world I would never have ventured to by myself.

My first journey abroad with the choir was in April 1987, touring the West Coast of America and Canada and I experienced my first flight at the age of 28. I should say that this trip would have been impossible for a wheelchair user (not that there were any in the choir at that time).

The choir gave concerts starting in California from San Francisco, then up through Sacramento, on to Portland in Oregon, then Seattle, and finally Vancouver in British Columbia.

We had the privilege of staying in the homes of people who were part of local choirs. This added an extra layer of significance to the tour, enabling us to experience the culture firsthand and life in the local communities we visited. We weren't just "tourists".

It was a remarkable trip. Each place has its own special aura and story lingering in my memory decades later and I could write much about the entire tour, but in short, I fell in love with San Francisco. I could have lived there in an instant and I spent four marvellous days there.

My lovely host, Trish, loved living there too, and she didn't hold back showcasing the many wonderful things about the city and local area. We embarked on a sensory adventure in Napa Valley, where we indulged in wine tasting at the exquisite Grgich Hills while basking in the scenic beauty that surrounded us. The aroma of the vineyards filled the air as we sat and relished a delightful picnic, savouring every moment of our experience.

Trish lived near San Rafael, and early one morning as we made our way towards the Golden Gate Bridge into the city centre, she parked up and we stepped out to look at the view. I wasn't prepared for the effect the scene would have on me.

32. MISTY

There before my eyes was one of the most beautiful sights I'd ever seen in all my born days. It took my breath away, and it took me completely by surprise: we were approaching a sprawling city, right? Hardly the place to be emotionally moved by the scenery.

The crimson peaks of the iconic Golden Gate Bridge were peeping above an expanse of fluffy, radiant clouds that were as white as snow. On the far horizon was a mirage of the shimmering sea, the colour of gold, intercepted by the city's striking geometric skyline.

An enormous lump came to my throat, and my eyes misted up.

I wasn't expecting that.

It was inexplicable.

Maybe it was because the vista combined a powerful fusion of human ingenuity with the natural splendour of the morning mist. I still do not know.

What I do know is that as the choir assembled in the Davies Symphony Hall for the next four evenings to perform Beethoven's 9th Symphony with the San Francisco Symphony Orchestra, the luscious 3rd movement vividly recreated the beauty of that scene in my mind every time. Under the talented baton of our conductor, Wolfgang Sawallisch, the sensitivity of his interpretation of this magical movement brought the lump into my throat yet again. Maybe he'd also witnessed the indescribable radiance of the mist, which had influenced how he conducted Beethoven's music with such poignant expression.

San Francisco had so much to savour - from clam chowders and discovering tasty Mexican food to colourful China Town, the joy of the hills and trams, seeing the world-famous prison Alcatraz in the distance and the thrill of shopping at Macy's, and to top it all off the busy-ness of the city. Trish was a wonderful tour guide, happy to taxi me around from place to place.

'What does ped zing mean?' I asked Trish as she drove through the city.

'Ped zing?' Trish double-checked.

'Yes, look, there it is! It's written all over the roads here,' I said, pointing at the two words as we pulled up at a pedestrian crossing.

PED

XING

Trish burst out laughing at my unthinkingness.

'It's short for pedestrian crossing!' she explained in fits of laughter.

Of course. Silly me!

I scratched my head at my stupidity.

Mind you, I didn't expect that walking the streets of San Francisco would cause me to wake up each morning dreaming about grids. I saw them in my sleep. I'd lived and grown up in the UK's second city, Birmingham, where the streets are all higgledy-piggledy with no rhyme nor reason to them, but in San Francisco, the streets are straight and logical in a marvellous grid system, unlike my hometown.

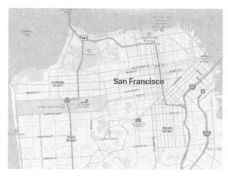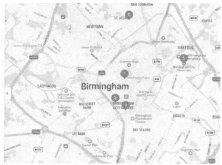

I messed up big time though with the gifts I bought for my six hosts. It was difficult to know what to buy them, but I wanted to give them something to show my appreciation for their hospitality—something small enough to take on a flight, but something which had value, something quintessentially English (don't all Americans like England?) and something useful yet also a keepsake. So I settled on a piece of Wedgwood China in the exquisite and delicate "Chinese Legend" design: an ashtray.

This was a big mistake.

Smoking was not in vogue in the States in the late eighties and was fast becoming socially unacceptable. I've never been a smoker myself, but I erroneously assumed every American would be.

None of my hosts were smokers.

My enchanting host Trish had made it plain as soon as I stepped over the threshold of her home that smoking was not allowed.

Needless to say, she was not impressed with my gift.

'An ashtray?' she remarked quizzically glancing sideways at me with a wry smile without malice, as she unwrapped her gift. *Oops.*

Thank you CBSO Chorus for a sensational travel experience. I've certainly left some of my heart in San Francisco. I hope I can visit again one day.

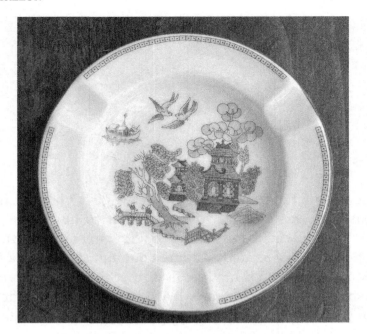

Wedgewood Chinese Legend Ashtray

33. CONTINENTAL CAPERS WITH THE CHOIR

More trips abroad followed with the CBSO Chorus. In March 1989, the choir did a short three-night tour in Belgium encompassing Antwerp, Ghent and Brussels, singing Mahler's Resurrection Symphony with the Royal Flanders Philharmonic Orchestra under the baton of Gunter Neuhold, who all the ladies thought was exceedingly handsome.

We boarded our flight, a Boeing 747, at 9.50 a.m. on Thursday, 16th of March 1989, and made a very bumpy ascent into the grey clouds. Penetrating cold and torrential rain greeted us when we landed in Brussels. Our coaches took us to the Hotel Arcade in Antwerp along the E19 autoroute through flat agricultural land, which was extremely waterlogged.

We experienced the cloudburst of the century just as the coach deposited us as far away as possible from the main entrance of Singel Hall for our first rehearsal. We all got soaking wet as we made a mad dash for the entrance.

'Crikey, the weather here's worse than in England!' we bemoaned.

What a bedraggled motley crew we must have looked at that first rehearsal.

'Where's the orchestra?' we wondered, as we got into our places.

They're late!

It was to become a pattern of behaviour—the Flanders Phil was consistently behind time for rehearsals. Thankfully, they turned up on time for the concerts.

St. Michael's Church in Ghent hosted our first concert, where we were packed like sardines with little room between the rows. Most of the choristers at the rear needed a head for heights, including me, as I was always at the back and on the end. The second row couldn't see the conductor, so they had to stand on their benches, resulting in the third row having to stand on their benches as well. We were perched precariously high on the planks.

Such is the life of a chorister.

Added to that, there was the additional hazard of singing almost bereft of oxygen because of the continuously burning calor gas heaters. They were great big things that looked like long-necked aliens with their heating element at the top of a four-foot pipe attached to the top of a cylinder. But they certainly tamed the bone-chilling March temperatures in the ancient church building.

'Where's the audience?' we wondered as we squashed together ready for the concert.

*Crikey, maybe nobody wants to come and hear the choir from Birmingham...*but the audience trickled in and we soon learned that Continental time differed from British time: it's perfectly acceptable for a concert to start at least 15 minutes late. All times are approximate!

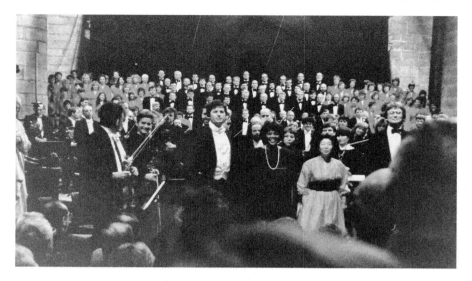

Concert in St Michael's Church, Ghent.
Left to right - Conductor - Gunter Neuhold
Contralto - Florence Quivar, Soprano - Mitsuko
Shirai, Chorus Master - Simon Halsey.
I'm the tallest one, right at the very back on the left-hand side.
(I loved our red dresses - we had to sew them
ourselves, made to a pattern.)

I fell in love with Ghent, a magnificent city even in the rain, and it's there I discovered things like *Kir Royales* and Ghent lace. Our hotel in Antwerp was opposite a delightful market, where we mooched the stalls; there were cheeses, sausages, flowers and fruit where the oranges were the size of grapefruits, along with Belgian lace and beautifully decorated Easter eggs amongst other treasures, both edible and inedible.

One tenor bought a marvellous sausage, which was over a foot long and nearly two inches in diameter. *Would British Customs impound it?* ...and then, of course, there was the amazing Rubens House with its glorious works of art by Rubens and Van Dyke, lovely stuff. As I gazed at the masterpieces painted in such detail, I couldn't help but compare them to the choir's art form of making music, which is so transient: music - once it's gone - it's gone. But these paintings would endure for centuries.

In Brussels, a group of us sopranos went on a mission to witness a display of male sexuality in the form of the *Manneken Pis.*

'Is that it?' questioned my friend as we stood staring up at a statue of a small boy-child peeing a long way down into a large basin. I'm not sure what we were expecting, but he sure was cute.

I'm happy to report that the tenor's sausage passed through British Customs with no problem. He was well pleased.

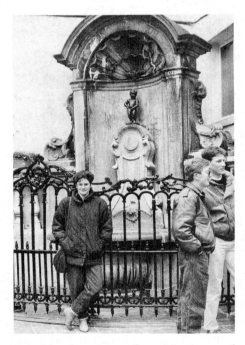

Outside the Manneken Pis, Brussels

34. VIVA ESPAÑA

Just over a year later in July 1990 the choir, along with our very own City of Birmingham Orchestra and conductor Simon Rattle (he wasn't a "Sir" then), flew off to Spain for a short tour in Madrid and Granada performing Beethoven's 9th Symphony.

We arrived mid-afternoon at Madrid Barajas Airport on Friday, 6th of July and transferred to Hotel Plaza, where we settled in and had the afternoon and evening free.

A relentless heatwave engulfed Madrid, causing the air to feel suffocatingly dry. The bustling streets echoed with the incessant noise of traffic, overwhelming my senses. The dusty pavements added to the gritty atmosphere of the city. Despite this, the main square offered respite, its spaciousness and elegance creating a serene oasis amidst the chaos.

Another highlight was savouring a Spanish meal on the first evening with several other choristers. Someone suggested we suss out a restaurant off the beaten track - somewhere the locals would eat and which would be a lot cheaper. So off we trekked and found a small place not frequented by tourists. It was simple, local food, and very cheap. I finished my tasty starter and put my knife and fork together on my empty plate, showing I was ready for the next course, but what happened next surprised me.

35. BUEN PROVECHO

The waitress took my cutlery off the plate and placed it back on the table, ready for the main meal. *Fair enough, it saves on the washing up, I guess.*

'*Buen provecho,*' she intoned as she placed my delicious main course in front of me between my dirty cutlery.

We were on a tight schedule from the next morning onwards, including a full orchestral rehearsal at *Palacio de Congresos.* We'd rehearsed singing the 4th movement of Beethoven's 9th Symphony, the famous "Ode to Joy", for many months, including the gentle and tender section *"Ihr stürzt nieder, Millionen!"* (Do you fall headlong, O millions?), but Maestro Simon Rattle was not happy with it.

'No, no, no, no, no,' he intoned, descending in pitch, 'that's just *so* bland, ladies and gentlemen. Please! You *must* sing it like…like…' we watched him as he searched for a poetic image to inveigle us to sing it with more expression '…to sing it like panting dogs, copulating.'

And so there we were, all genned up with that image in our minds, ready to deliver our amazing *Ihr stürzt nieder, Millionen!* and wow the Spaniards with our stunning singing, imitating panting dogs, copulating, at the appropriate moment.

Our orchestra assembled bang on time (unlike the Flanders Phil in Belgium who were consistently late) and we had a great rehearsal in a proper concert hall, with cushioned seats and air conditioning. All very civilised.

The soloists joining us included two of the world's most prestigious singers: bass-baritone Willard White, and tenor Robert Tear. We looked forward to the concert with anticipation. What a treat.

'Where's the audience?' we wondered *déjà vu* as the 8.00 p.m. scheduled start passed by, as did 8.15 p.m. and the auditorium was only half full. *But of course, we're on the Continent! All times are approximate.* We discovered that Spanish time is even later than Belgian time.

At least we didn't have to squish together and balance on planks this time. We each had our own cushioned seat in the concert hall with lots of legroom, and a good job too, as one of the tenors in the back row got up and left the stage in haste during the performance.

What's up with him?

No one batted an eyelid as if it happened at every concert, and then we hear him throw up backstage. He made it just in time.

'I think it was a bad mussel I ate earlier on,' he bemoaned. We congratulated him for being brave enough to walk off the concert platform. It would have been terribly bad if he'd thrown up all over the first sopranos.

I didn't connect with Madrid particularly. The rather basic hotel room with a tiny window did not help. In addition to that, they advised us to use bottled water at all times - even when cleaning our teeth - because it wasn't safe to use tap water in case it upset our delicate Brit tummies. I was glad when we moved on to Granada.

36. MEMORIES OF THE ALHAMBRA

On Sunday, the 8th of July, we were off bright and early at 8.15 a.m. for the short flight from Madrid to Granada. From the moment we touched down, the enchanting surrounding enraptured me. Together, our group ventured into a bustling local craft market, teeming with vibrant colours and lively chatter. Mooching through the stalls, I was infatuated with the array of exquisite pottery. I bought many pieces, each radiating exotic designs in brilliant hues.

We were all wonderfully excited about our visit to Granada because later that evening we would perform Beethoven's 9th Symphony at an outdoor concert on the exquisite grounds of the Alhambra Palace.

Was this really happening to me?

Singing with a world-class orchestra, with world-class soloists, under the baton of the renowned world-class conductor Simon Rattle, in the Alhambra Palace. Oh wow! This would be a unique and unforgettable experience.

How many choristers get to experience *that?!*

They scheduled our concert to start late at 10.00 p.m. This is not a time a British choir is used to, and in the UK our concerts are all over and done with by then and we're usually on our way home to get tucked up in bed. The reason for this ungodly start time, we were told, was because it was the night of the World Cup Final between Germany and Argentina. *Of course!* Football is far more important than an open-air concert in the Alhambra Palace. Beethoven is no match for the World Cup

Final.

Spain was enthralled with World Cup mania.

But first, we had a full orchestral rehearsal starting at 8.00 p.m. which we were not well pleased about as we'd all be knackered and sung out having to sing it all again later that same night, but we were up for the challenge and told ourselves we weren't made of sugar.

We'd get through it.

It was a beautifully warm, balmy evening - just perfect for an open-air concert.

And so the orchestra and choir duly assembled, ready to begin the concert at 10.00 p.m. prompt.

'Where's the audience?' we wondered as time dragged on and on.

And on.

In Britain, we ALWAYS start concerts bang on time. But our Spanish audience was nowhere to be seen.

10.15 p.m. Not a soul.

10.30 p.m. Still deserted. Not a single bum on seat.

Where the heck is everyone? They've bought the tickets. It's a sell-out!

10.45 p.m. At last! The audience trickled in. By this time we'd been waiting around nearly an hour, and we were all getting rather pigged off, especially the choir (and probably the poor soloists as well) as we wouldn't be singing for another hour because the orchestra had to play the first three movements before we even sang a note.

After a few more minutes, the punters were all seated and ready, unperturbed by their lateness.

The orchestra began, and we just sat and listened for an hour as they strutted their stuff for the first three movements. My bum was feeling sore from the hard seat. Then it was our turn.

Finally!

Our Maestro gestured to us to stand, and we arose as one body ready to sing the famous fourth movement, *"Ode to Joy."*

By now, it's nearly midnight.

'Bloody hell, what was that?' whispered my fellow soprano, frantic with fear as something black whizzed passed by our heads.

We froze.

37. STIFF UPPER LIP IN SPAIN

'It's a bat!!' I whispered back as another one swooped over us and I resisted a powerful urge to duck.

'Shit! I hate them!' she hissed, just as the angry and turbulent chords of the 4th movement began like a portent of doom as another bat flew past us, and then another and another.

Soon there was a colony of bats flying erratically around the choir and orchestra. We had to suppress the urge to shoo them away and run.

It didn't take long to realise that the bats were quite harmless and not going to attack us.

The show must go on!

And go on it did, with the bats gracefully flitting through the air like skilled aerial gymnasts, dancing in perfect harmony with the melodies of our music, which were carried into the vast expanse of the ether.

As the night wore on, the concert reached its crescendo and enveloped the surroundings with an atmosphere of electrifying energy while the audience basked in the enchanting ambience. Finally, as the clock struck midnight and the last notes reverberated through the night, an echo of awe and satisfaction filled both the audience and musicians alike.

However, our Maestro was not well pleased with World Cup lateness.

Thank you again, CBSO Chorus, for a magnificent choral experience abroad. I am truly grateful.

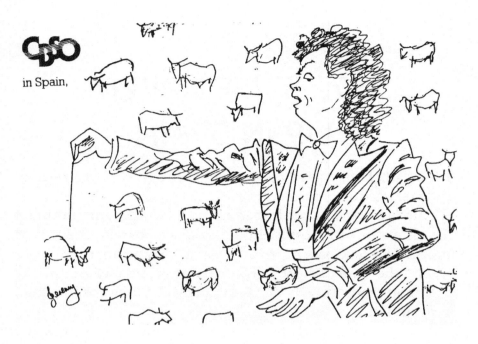

CARTOON OF SIMON RATTLE in Spain
by Jeremy Ballard (Leader of the 2nd fiddles)
By kind permission of the Ballard Family

PART FOUR - SWISS FAMILY FALLON

38. ALPINE ASPIRATIONS

When I moved to Devon and married Don in 1994, I accepted that I probably wouldn't ever travel abroad again, resigned to the fact that my flying days were over.

But they weren't quite.

I had one flight coming my way, albeit on my own.

Ever since our holiday in the French Alps, we'd longed to visit Switzerland and witness the majestic mountains there. There is an indescribable allure to these snowy peaks, captivating us with their awe-inspiring beauty and majestic presence. The sight of the mountains, adorned with a pristine blanket of glistening snow, offers a unique perspective on life, evoking a profound sense of wonder and contemplation. The crisp, pure air carries a hint of freshness, invigorating the senses and rejuvenating the soul. This tranquil setting, however, is not devoid of life and prosperity. The thriving economy manifests itself in the impeccable quality of the amenities and infrastructure that surround these mountains, a testament to the wealth they generate.

So we were overjoyed when Don came across a two-week "Swiss family holiday" in a large chalet with several other families. It would be communal living where we would all pitch in with preparing food, cooking and washing up. Not really my thing, though it was cheap and an ideal way to see the sights of the Alps.

But we have a bit of a dilemma.

39. SWITZERLAND 2007

The holiday is in just a few months and the first week coincides with a singing course that I've paid for at Dartington International Summer School, near the quirky town of Totnes. I won't get any refund if I cancel my singing course, so Don and Tim will drive to Switzerland without me. I'll fly out after finishing my course and join them for the second week. So Don goes ahead and books it all up, car ferry and all.

Don is now using a manual wheelchair. He'd had a series of falls a few years previously where one of his knees kept collapsing, and he'd also put on some weight. Walking in callipers with a walking stick had become a liability, so a wheelchair was safer and an ideal solution. He could whiz around the bungalow in it with no problem at all. We also switched our car to a Toyota Yaris, which allowed us to load the folding wheelchair more easily into the boot.

Don and Tim have a pleasant journey driving out to Switzerland and they settle in well with all the friendly families in the chalet. I am going to fly out to Geneva Airport where Don will meet me.

I spent an exhilarating week singing in the Summer School Choir, culminating in a glorious concert of William Walton's *Belshazzar's Feast* conducted by Bob Chilcott in the amazing Dartington Hall.

We now also have a beautiful Cavalier King Charles Spaniel —Sam. Tim had written several letters to us asking for a dog, so we relented. But what to do with our pooch while we are abroad? Through an internet search, I discovered an organisation called "Pet Sitter Swap" so I registered with them and found that there's a local couple who agreed to look after our Sammy.

We also now have four tropical fish tanks with African Cichlids in them. It's a new hobby which keeps me busy cleaning the tanks out every few weeks. The fish have been breeding and because cichlids are territorial and will fight, they had to be split up into separate tanks.

I'm fascinated by the vivid and vibrant colours of our African Cichlids and mesmerised by observing the mother fish cradle her offspring in her mouth. She spits the fry out when it is safe, and quickly sucks them back in at the first sign of danger. It's like watching a miracle.

I arrange for Tim's friend, Ashley, to assist with feeding the fish while we are abroad. Every summer, Ashley stays with his grandparents - Peter and Betty - who live a few doors away, and he's a keen and willing helper. I show him how to feed the fish and give him a key to let himself into our bungalow. Then, after dropping Sam at Hayley's, I pack and head to the coach taking me to Heathrow Airport.

While I'm at the airport, I get a text message from Don (which must have taken him half an hour to write - despite his lack of punctuation - as he simply will NOT use predictive text).

Great news darling I've met a wonderful couple called Steph and Rob and they have a hotel in Switzerland Rob has kindly offered to come and pick you up from Geneva airport and drive you to the chalet so that me and Tim can go up the Jungfraujoch Rob does airport runs all the time for his guests he's used to it he'll be holding up a board with your name on it love Don XX

I board the British Airways plane on time, but then it goes nowhere. Two hours later, all the passengers are still sitting on a stationary plane which is grounded for no apparent reason. Then, as if nothing had happened, the plane taxis onto the runway and we're off.

On arrival at Geneva Airport, sure enough, I see my name 'DAWN' on a placard held high, which makes me feel rather important. Rob is very good about the two-hour wait and explains that he's used to flights being delayed, but putting myself in his shoes, I'd have felt miffed. I keep apologising even though it isn't my fault. It's late in the evening when I get to the chalet, and this timing is bad for me because I'd had a slight hiccup at Heathrow Airport, which caused me a bit of a problem.

40. FLUID RESTRICTIONS

The culprit was my contact lens fluid. In 2006, there had been a terrorist plot to detonate liquid explosives on planes travelling from the United Kingdom to the United States and Canada, disguised as soft drinks. All UK airlines were operating extra vigilance about any fluids.

British Airways had wanted to confiscate my 200ml bottle of contact lens solution. I'm unaware that there is a limit of 100ml on all fluids and I only learned about this at the airport. If only I'd bought a smaller bottle, it would have been fine. I explained that I desperately needed the fluid for medical reasons and that my contact lenses had to be soaked overnight in the solution or they would dry out.

They allowed me to wrap it in a plastic bag and promised it would be ready and waiting in Switzerland.

But it never arrived[1].

Surely this couldn't have been the reason for the two-hour delay?

Even though Rob had been waiting for an extra two hours, he patiently waited a little longer to see if my bottle of liquid would turn up, but I doubt it had ever left the UK.

All the chemists were closed by the time I arrived in Geneva and I'd have to wait until the morning to buy some new fluid.

I arrive at the chalet and it's good to see Don and Tim again. Over a late-night snack and cocoa, I'm introduced to all the lovely families there, and I'm very proud of our Tim (now 13 years old) who I'm told has been doing his share of food prep and washing up duties. Everyone comments on how helpful he is.

I have no choice but to sleep in my contact lenses. The problem is that they are not the special kind for sleeping in, so the next morning my eyes are stuck together. I splash them with water and prise them open, but they are dry and sore and in a bad way.

After a quick breakfast, we are off to the nearest village to find a *Pharmacie* and I'm soon back to normal with some lubricating eye drops after the lenses have soaked a while in their special juice.

Later that evening, we gather around the spacious outdoor table, with flickering candlelight creating a cosy ambience. We indulge in a traditional Swiss dish and enjoy a fun fondue feast, dipping our bread into melted cheese and wine. The clinking of forks against the communal pot and the laughter of friends intertwine, creating a fusion of merriment. Mind you, I'm shocked at how boozy this Swiss dish is. No wonder fondue was a thing back in the seventies. What a perfect meal to share with friends in a Swiss chalet in Switzerland!

After supper, we play a ball game on the lawn. Don, being Don, doesn't want to miss out on anything. He follows everyone down the grassy slope to join the game. However, his wheels get stuck in the soft grass when he tries to return to the patio area. It takes four men to lift him and his chair back onto solid ground. He's politely banned from going down to the lawn for the rest of the week.

[1] *On return home I complain to British Airways and get a full refund of my fare.*

41. A DREAM COME TRUE

Tim and Don had a wonderful week without me.

'We had a marvellous tour up the Jungfraujoch mountain,' Don enthused. 'It's a pity you missed that outing. You should've seen them transfer me from one train to another on a forklift truck! It was terrific. Tim went snowboarding when we reached the top, but he got a bout of mountain sickness later.'

'Oh no, what's that? Was he all right?'

'He had a headache and was a bit dizzy for a while, but it soon passed. Tim was hoping to go on a sled ride, but it was too hot for the Huskies. They were all wilting.'

'A sled ride? With dogs?' I perk up. 'I'd absolutely love that!'

I'd long had a fantasy of travelling through snow at high speed. I loved the dinky Christmas song "Jingle Bells", especially the verse *"Dashing through the snow in a one-horse open sleigh, o'er the hills we go, laughing all the way."* I could just picture the scene with fresh cold air kissing the cheeks, fine morsels of snow dusting the face, and the thrill of velocity, but I'd never thought it would ever be possible. Except this would be with dogs, not horses.

'Well, it might be possible darling when we go to Glacier 3000. It's on our itinerary as part of the Swiss family holiday. That's if the Huskies aren't too hot.'

So, travelling at speed through the snow was now within my reach. At last, my fantasy was about to be realised.

We arrive at Glacier 3000, but something's not right.

42. GLACIER 3000

First, there is no "*glace*".

There's no ice and no snow.

Just grey dirt.

Déjà vu Glace de Mer at Mont Blanc.

It's so hot that I walk on the glacier in my flip-flops (and it's not a good idea as it's quite stony and makes treading on it difficult. Do I never learn?). I get some strange looks.

There isn't a cat's chance in hell of a sled ride with the dogs because of the heat, quite apart from the fact that dog-sled rides need to be pre-booked, and we hadn't pre-booked anything.

'But there's a toboggan ride called the Alpine Coaster,' advises the assistant, having witnessed my disappointment. 'It's the highest toboggan ride in the world,' he boasts.

'Oh great, well I'll have a go on that then instead with my son. Two tickets, please.'

The ride looks like a toddler's version of the "big dipper" and there's no snow to be seen anywhere. I have to resist the urge to laugh as it's a picture of incongruity. *A toboggan ride over grey, dusty dirt?* It's a rather sad sight and the toboggan, laid bare on its supporting frame, looks like a giant *Meccano* construction. At least Tim is enjoying it all, snow or no snow.

Even though I'm prone to daydreaming, my imagination just can't make it feel as if I am whizzing through soft, flaky snow. The sun is hot, and my face is wind burnt. Still, I love being immersed in the velocity. We give it some welly and whizz along at every twist and turn. It *is* rather fun!

The ride comes to a halt and I grab the sides to lift myself out.

But there's a complication. In fact, there are two complications.

43. TROUBLE AT T'MILL

The first is that I can't move. The twists and turns at speed on the toboggan ride have put my back out. I had felt no pain during the joyride, but now it's kicking in. I take some deep breaths and, in slow motion, I prise myself from the seat and hobble to our car.

At the chalet I rest, dosed up with paracetamol. After a good night's sleep, my back settles down and the next morning, the pain has passed. I have a lucky escape. It could have been so much worse.

Then my mobile rings.

'Hello Dawn, it's Betty here,' says Ashley's grandma.

Oh crikey, have all the fish died?

'Our Ash has locked himself out of your bungalow!' she wails in her Birmingham accent, which is even stronger than mine (there are a lot of us Brummies in Torbay).

'Well, we're coming home soon, Betty, so please don't worry,' I soothe.

'But the key is on the inside of the front door!'

Oh.

Now, that *is* bad news.

It means we can't open the door if he's left the spare key in the lock.

How the hell did he lock himself out, leaving the key in the door on the inside?

We have no side entrance to our bungalow, and all the keys

to the patio doors are in the keyholes.

We are well and truly locked out.

'Ashley's very upset,' Betty explains. 'He put the key in the lock inside so that he wouldn't lose it, but the door blew shut when he went outside to fetch a parcel and he can't get back in!'

'Please don't worry Betty and tell Ashley not to worry.'

'He's too young to have had all that responsibility for feeding the fish put on him,' she bemoans.

'I'm so sorry, but I promise we'll sort something out and I'll ring you back.'

But it is a problem. We will arrive home late at night and there's no way we can break into our own property. It demands a drastic solution. With much effort, my mobile phone bill mounting with dozens of calls, I arrange for a glazier in Brixham to take out our kitchen window, retrieve the key, and then put the window back.

The plan works.

Forty-eight hours later, the glazing company has done their magic, and the key is in Betty's hands for safekeeping until we return.

Our time in Switzerland is coming to an end, and the beauty of the country has moved us. We visit Château-d'Oex in Rougement on our way home, and Don discovers that disabled people can do armchair skiing during the winter months. This excites Don tremendously. He's a fan of watching the TV programme Ski Sunday where the skiers fly down the hills at almost 100 mph.

'They're nutters!' I said, declaring my verdict on the speed the skiers plummet down the snowy slopes.

'I know. They're crazy,' responds Don. 'But I'd love to do it.'

However, the pursuit of armchair skiing is still on his "bucket list" of things to do as he's never made it back to Chamonix to try it.

It's strange: although Don refuses to fly in a plane, when it comes to extreme sports, he doesn't give a toss about the danger of death; he has sailed jibs adapted for the disabled and he rides a handcycle on roads around Devon where he was almost sandwiched between a bus and car, and nearly run into by a lorry, but it still doesn't stop him. It makes little sense, but there we are.

We savour every last picking of France that we can on our long drive home, detouring to Quimper where Tim experiences his very first *moules marinière.* Don is wary of mollusc-type foods, and mussels remind me of my 1960s childhood when my father would boil them up filling the house with their stench, then eat them cold seasoned with salt, pepper and vinegar. I wasn't a fan. So we plump for a traditional *coq au vin* dish. But Tim has no such inhibitions and is blown away by his choice as he savours the enticing *moules marinière*, served with crunchy *frites* and a delectable crusty baguette to mop up the juices. The plump, succulent mussels bathe in a fragrant creamy broth, and the gentle aroma of garlic, white wine, and fresh herbs arrest his senses with the tantalising harmonious flavours of the briny sea. This culinary delight is a revelation to Tim, and it becomes one of his favourite dishes to order when on the menu in any restaurant at home or abroad.

I loved our chalet in Switzerland; it was so pretty. The peace and serenity of the place will stay with me for always, especially looking out of our bedroom window each morning and seeing the cows, and hearing the soothing sound of the gentle tinkling bells around their necks.

What an idyll.

Thank you, Switzerland, for a little bit of heaven on earth.

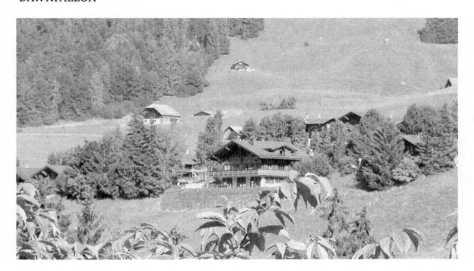

The "Swiss Family Holiday" chalet

PART FIVE - CRUISING CAPERS

44. MEDITERRANEAN MEANDERINGS - 2008

Soon after our Swiss Family Holiday in 2007, we visit the Wiltshire County Show. Tim is into keeping gerbils and Don, in his inimitable way, is not content for Tim to have just one gerbil. Oh no, he's got ten of them, all in various colours. A veritable rodent-fest.

So off we toddle, complete with several of Tim's gerbils in tow, one of which wins First Prize when Lulu, a Roborovsky, charms the judges, and Tim of course is over the moon.

Don gets ripped off when he pays £200 for a home massage set (which ends up unused in the loft), but otherwise, the show is enjoyable overall.

We wind up at a stand for "Disabled and Accessible Travel," where the assistant talks us into booking a 10-night Mediterranean cruise.

'You'll love it!' she enthuses. 'You won't regret it. It'll be the perfect family holiday.'

She assures us we'll have an accessible cabin onboard the Royal Caribbean's brand-spanking-new cruise liner *Independence of the Seas* for its maiden voyage, no less, in August 2008. Because Don won't fly, travelling with him to faraway places is challenging, so a cruise presents a wonderful way to explore the globe.

We splash out on this venture and book an inside cabin -

no windows, not even a porthole. Nonetheless, I am excited. A maiden voyage! *Hope it doesn't sink like the Titanic.*

From the brochure, I discover the ship is colossal, with an ice rink, surf machine, climbing wall and two superb whirlpools which hang over the sides of the vessel. What a treat. And we get an extra perk of free parking at the Port of Southampton for the full ten days. We will dine at the luxurious King Lear Restaurant, which boasts excellent food.

Early in 2008, we receive a letter from Royal Caribbean about what to pack for the cruise, and we are completely unprepared for one of their commands.

45. THE CRUISE AND THE COCKTAIL DRESS

The cruise line instructs us to bring some formal evening wear, including full evening dress for men, and cocktail dresses for women. This dress code is required for the occasional "formal" evenings in the King Lear Restaurant.

I've never owned or worn a cocktail dress in my life. I go hunting for one in all the charity shops in Torquay and find a slinky number I quite like and try it on, though it's not an easy garment to get into as it's a tight fit. My middle-age spread is showing, and I decide I look ghastly in it. I attempt to take it off and I get stuck trying to pull the garment off over my head.

'Excuse me!' I shout to the shop assistant from the changing room, with my arms trapped up in the air and the garment over my head. 'Can you help me, please?'

The assistant comes and helps to peel it off my body. *Good job it's not a bloke!*

I play it safe in the end and buy a new frock in a sale at Marks and Spencer, though it's not strictly a cocktail dress. But who would notice? It will have to do. Tim and Don decide to wing it with a smart jacket over some flannels (or in Tim's case, stylish jeans).

46. PRIMROSE

Don now also has an electric wheelchair for outdoor use as well as his manual wheelchair, which he uses inside the bungalow.

I was finding pushing him up hills in his manual wheelchair a struggle, especially as he has put on more weight. Even though he has a lot of upper body strength, it's tiring for him to wheel himself, so the electric wheelchair is a fantastic asset. But it wouldn't go into our Toyota Yaris car, so we had to invest in a much larger vehicle to accommodate the electric wheelchair.

If you're disabled and want to enjoy a comfortable standard of mobility, it can't be done on the cheap, so we'd re-mortgaged our bungalow enabling Don to purchase a Mercedes Sprinter van with a high roof and fitted with a wheelchair lift.

I couldn't help but give our new Mercedes a name - Primrose. Such a dainty title for a colossal vehicle. I loved the incongruity.

Don meticulously researched the type of van and wheelchair lift that would be best for him and his needs. It's not as easy as it sounds and for several months we traipsed around the country trying out several secondhand accessible vehicles, but they were all completely unsuitable. So a brand new vehicle, which would tick all the boxes, was the best - and in the end the cheapest - solution. It would last for many years.

The high roof in Primrose also meant that Don, who was over six feet tall, didn't have to bend his neck at an uncomfortable angle every time he wanted to get in and out of the van. The wheelchair lift he chose, a "Braun" made in the

USA, was ingenious. It came out neatly at the side and, once lowered to ground level, he wheeled himself onto it then lifted him and backed him into the van. This meant he didn't have to enter the vehicle on a long ramp from the side or through the rear.

The cost was eye-watering for us, though, and we could have bought a small house for what we paid for Primrose. But she gave us so much more freedom to travel, and it meant that Don was now independent. He could get in and out of the van himself without my help, and transfer to the driver's seat.

Despite her size, Primrose is very easy to drive with her power steering, and she is automatic. Don has hand controls fitted, but I can drive Primrose too, like a normal van. And yes, you've guessed it, I pranged our van on the second day after we got it, no less. I'd dropped Tim off at school and misjudged the width of Primrose, putting a small dent in the door when I caught the wing mirror of a parked car. The owner of the car was not well pleased, but we sorted it out on the insurance, and our van had to have bodywork to restore it.

The day before we leave for the cruise, I get out my "Holiday List" (I love my lists) to make sure I haven't forgotten anything:

Cruise Ship Tickets - Tick
Insurance papers - Tick
Passports - Tick
EU Health Cards - Tick
200 Euros cash - Tick
Envelopes with dollars in for our "gratuities" - Tick

We're good to go.

On the 27th of August 2008, we set off early from Brixham in Primrose the van and arrive at the Port of Southampton where we drop off our huge amount of luggage for the porters to take care of, then we park up in the allotted disabled space. After checking in and boarding the ship, we find our cabin and it has a little surprise for us.

47. THE CABIN
(...oh, sorry, I mean the "Stateroom")

We are greeted by a creature on our bed. *So cute!*

Our wonderful Filipino room attendant, Aniceto, made it from a towel. This art form is like origami but uses towels rather than paper. We think it is rather clever. The exact originator of towel animals is unknown, but they are popular in many cruise lines and high-end hotels. Well, I guess "little things please little minds" might be an observer's thought, but it is one of the small things that makes you feel good and enraptures young Tim.

We love the smart cabin and spacious, accessible bathroom. I do not like rooms without windows, but on our budget, it was an inside cabin or nothing at all. I can live with it. We will only be using it to sleep and get changed in.

'What's the bed like?' enquires Don.

I always expect this question every time we go away, as I'm the bed-trier-outer. I flop down onto it, not hopeful that it will be to his liking (they never are), but I'm pleasantly surprised.

'It's fantastic! You'll love it! It's soft but supportive. How did they manage that?'

Don is "thinly upholstered" (as he describes it) on his hips and buttocks because of his disability and is prone to bedsores, so a soft, yet supportive, mattress is essential for medical reasons (let alone his personal comfort). Just another issue to be sorted on travels when the beds are firm and an extra duvet to lie on has to be called for - but not on this occasion. Tim has a bunk bed, and bunks are always fun for young teens.

◆ ◆ ◆

We go off and explore some of the ship and we're intrigued by the size of it. The *Independence of the Seas* can accommodate over 5,000 passengers and crew and has over 15 decks. The ship is HUGE! It's like a small floating city. Don's vertigo is getting a little better, but he still feels queasy in the lifts. They are all mirror and glass and from the top deck 14, you can see right down to the bottom deck. I feel a tad queasy in them myself. What if the cables break? It didn't bear thinking about.

We set sail, though it turns out our trip was not the ship's maiden voyage after all, as it had already set sail on the 2nd of May, 2008. Either the sales rep lied to us, or the cruise line got their facts wrong. But never mind, it is still a very swanky brand-new ship.

Don's mind is consumed with worry as he contemplates crossing the treacherous Bay of Biscay.

'I don't want to be seasick,' he frets.

I conclude he's faking it. He needn't have worried - the Bay of Biscay behaves very well and we have a smooth crossing.

I'm enamoured by the peculiar *objets d'art,* pictures and paintings scattered around the various decks onboard. Bright red giant plastic dogs, blue plastic sheep, and intriguing images line every deck.

We find the sheer number of passengers to be overwhelming. It's a busy, bustling ship, especially when we hit warmer climes and we find we can't get a deck chair for love or money. It's packed. Talk about catering for the masses.

From dawn until the early hours, the life on board ship is constant. Food is super-abundant, and we can't eat all that is on offer, though some passengers seem to have no problem stuffing their faces all day, and we wonder where they put it all.

… But land is looming - our first port of call - and I can't wait to get a mobile phone signal. I have an urgent call to make.

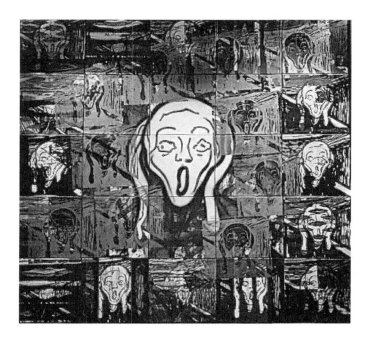

*Based on "The Scream" - an artwork made from
tiles on board Independence of the Seas,
I wasn't a fan of it.*

48. FIRST STOP - GIBRALTAR

As soon as I'm in port, I call my Turkish friend Elif, who lives in Brixham, because she and her English husband are looking after our pooch, Sam.

'Hi Elif! How's Sam? Is he behaving himself?'

'Don't worry! Don't worry! He is fine. He's eating an apple. Just enjoy your holiday, OK?' she assures me.

Eating an apple?

I know our dog has an ENORMOUS appetite, but I've never seen him eat any fruit. *Oh well, he must be happy then.*

Reassured, I head straight for a small pop-up stall in the corner of the plaza selling watches for £5 and buy three of them. *So many to choose from.*

We head off down the main drag to find a cold lager.

'Be careful crossing the roads, they drive on the right even though Gibraltar is British,' observes Don, 'and you'll never guess which famous couple got married here?'

'Er, I've no idea. Enlighten me.'

'Take a guess.'

'Oh, I don't know, erm, Posh and Becks?'

'John Lennon and Yoko Ono. You can get married within 24 hours once you lodge your papers here. How's that for efficiency?'

'Impressive.'

As we approach the town centre, there are rows of derelict cars covered in dust. *I wonder why?* A Celtic football fan had taken a shine to one of them, writing in the dust on the windscreen. It seemed out of kilter with the efficiency of speed a couple can get married there.

We relish a delightful time on The Rock, where the vibrant colours and fragrant scents of the Botanical Gardens stimulate our senses. As we navigate through, we skilfully dodge the mischievous monkeys who attempt to snatch our belongings. Afterwards, we indulge in a delectable light lunch at one of the many bars, savouring the local flavours and beers.

After browsing the many shops where Don buys a superb camera, we head back to the ship for our evening meal. While Don and Tim grab a game of Shuffleboard on Deck 4, I learn an interesting fact about this incredible vessel.

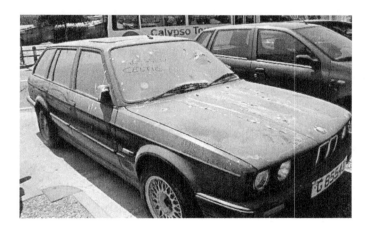

One of the many dusty, derelict cars in Gibraltar.
A Celtic fan took a shine to this one!

49. POOP DECK

I discover that the *Independence of the Seas* has no poop deck - not that this is particularly concerning or of any great importance - but it's a nautical fact I find fascinating.

The poop deck has nothing to do with poop mind, and sailors did not use it to relieve themselves. Rather, in the past, it used to be an important part of the ship design, being located at a high point for observational purposes. The Titanic was one of the last ships to have a traditional poop deck.

But what a strange name for an observational deck. One theory is that it's from the French word *"la poupe"* meaning "the stern" seeing as the poop deck was always at the rear of the ship.

Mind you, on the subject of poop, when disabled people get together, they often share their bladder and bowel troubles, comparing notes and exploring toileting solutions. Modern technology has now improved such difficulties for many disabled people, but at the time of our cruise, Don was prone to blocking toilets.

'What's that smell?' I ask Don as I walk into our cabin to get ready for dinner after a swim.

'I've had an accident,' he says.

Oh gawd, those words fill me with dread.

'Oh no, what's happened?'

'I went to the loo, and the pan got blocked,' he explains, 'but it's all been sorted.'

Thank God for that!

Don has a neuropathic bladder and bowel because of his disability, and bowel movements can be like the Number 43 bus - there are none for a while, and then three all come at once. I'd found my inner nurse being a carer for Don and had decided that the bottom line of nursing was dealing with bodily fluids, but it could be challenging. Don now uses a technique called bowel irrigation, which is also used by paralympic athletes, so this wouldn't happen to him today.

I'm thankful I wasn't there when he requested help, as I sometimes find such things embarrassing. The water in the lavatory pan had risen to the brim, Don said, and would not go down. A merry band of Filipino toilet technicians came and sorted it out, not batting an eyelid at the gory task. They are my heroes.

'They were wonderful,' says Don. 'They didn't seem to mind at all. Nothing was too much trouble for them.' *Well, they might have minded a lot but were too polite to say, I guess we'll never know.*

We go off to dinner.

We're not keen on the self-service restaurants. Why choose self-service when we can have someone wait on us? So we always opt to dine in the King Lear restaurant every day for breakfast, lunch and dinner. The downside is that it means queuing because there is a strict seating protocol, so it feels a bit like being back at school and getting in line for dinner. The restaurant is humungous, comprising three floors, with gigantic chandeliers dangling precariously from the vaulted ceiling. My jaw dropped in astonishment that the weight didn't cause the entire thing to come crashing down on the diners below.

After a lovely evening meal, we stroll around the deck at dusk and discover three illuminated swimming pools - an adult pool, a mixed-age pool and a children's pool. Needless to say, I ban Don from getting into the kiddies' pool.

Although we're stuffed from our evening meal, it's not long until there's a "sail away party" and the deck is rocking and heaving with all the cruise revellers drinking, dancing and eating (again). I'm flabbergasted at the amount of extravagant party food the ship's crew put on - not only the quantity but also the magnificent artistic creations they present. It looks too good to eat.

Next stop - Spain!

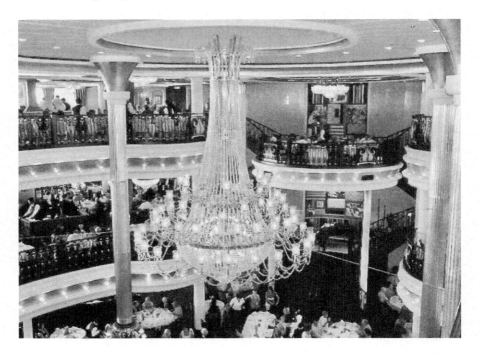

Chandelier in the King Lear Restaurant

50. BARCELONA

As I step out at the sunny port of Barcelona, Freddie Mercury's famous song about this venue is running through my head. The luscious lyrics speak of Barcelona's beautiful horizons, shining like a jewel in the sun. A place where you can become one of its lifelong friends. The words fill me with hope for my encounter with this fascinating city.

During the 1992 Olympics in Barcelona, Freddie and Montserrat Caballé made the song famous by performing it as a duet.

Caballé, a trained opera singer, was born in Barcelona in 1933 and her performance of this song with rock star Freddie Mercury in 1987 was pure genius. What a concept. A fusion of two amazing voices from opposite poles of the musical spectrum - it's one of my all-time favourite songs with the soaring soprano voice of Caballé contrasted against the versatile voice of Freddie Mercury.

Florid, powerful and unique, it reaches orgasmic proportions as the song builds to a climax.

It's a masterpiece.

I'm looking forward to Barcelona. Mind you, we decide to give the *Museu de l'Eròtica* which features a giant penis, a miss.

After marvelling at the mullet swimming in the harbour (Don and Tim are very much into their fishing and wish they'd got some tackle), we head for *Las Ramblas*, a once foul-smelling sewer street in Barcelona, but now a tree-lined boulevard full of kiosks, fragrant flower stalls, souvenir shops, bars, cafes, and many street performers strutting their stuff. It reminds me of a circus, except that I'm not a spectator, I'm part of the show right in the middle of it all. It's crowded and busy with tourists and sellers. We pause under the shade of an umbrella at a bar to savour a refreshing sangria which arrives in a glass the size of a small goldfish bowl. With three straws in hand, we share the fruity concoction, relishing its sweet and tangy flavours.

We find *Las Ramblas* somewhat chaotic and a tad overwhelming, so we about turn and retrace our steps back to the harbour, particularly as it's so hot and sticky. There's more space there with fewer people. We're afraid to go too far afield in case we get lost and miss the ship when it sets sail. Two passengers got left behind in Gibraltar because they were late and the ship can't wait for tardy passengers - the mooring fee charges are very expensive. So we kill time not too far from the dock in *Plaça Catalunya*. Tim and Don wander off to buy ice-cold bottled water, and I take a walk to the water's edge. But then, out of nowhere, I find myself surrounded.

51. THERE'S ALWAYS ONE...

A vast group of children are chattering at me in Spanish. One of them - a young girl - has a clipboard with names and numbers written in boxes along with a picture of a wheelchair at the top. *Aww, they must have seen me with Don earlier.*

'Petition! Petition!' she keeps saying, shoving the clipboard in my face.

She gives me the clipboard and wields a pen so that I can sign the "petition" and makes it plain she wants a donation for the "charity". I get out my purse and give them one euro just to get rid of them and stop them hassling me.

It works.

As soon as I hand over my euro and put my purse away, there's a rapid disassembly of the group and they vanish.

How strange.

Have I just dreamt that happened?

I'm standing alone at the water's edge.

I can't see Don and Tim anywhere, so I toddle off to the boutiques on the quay, browsing the souvenirs. They're a little more upmarket and not as tacky as some of the shops in *Las Ramblas*.

I notice an array of beautiful Spanish fans. *My, how I need one of those! It's so hot.* I choose a floral design and dip in my handbag for my purse.

But it's not there.

I feel stupid as I look and look.

But there's no purse.

It's gone.

Gone with the skilful pickpocket who'd nabbed it just as I'd put it back in my bag and I hadn't even felt it go. How clever! Inside my purse was two hundred euros cash, also gone in a flash, as well as our credit card and our boarding passes.

Stupid me, what a sucker! Trust me to be the 'one' the children were touting for—an inexperienced tourist, trusting and gullible.

Feeling concerned and alienated, I look for Don and Tim to tell them what's happened, but they're nowhere to be seen. I wander into the police station nearby in *Plaça Catalunya*. The children had robbed me right in front of the cops, the cheeky blighters! But the *policía* aren't interested and couldn't care less. They can do nothing about it.

As I meander back out into *Plaça Catalunya* Don and Tim are there. They're sad for me when I tell them my misfortune and take the news well.

'It means we've got no cash now for the rest of the cruise, and I can't draw any cash out because the credit card was in my purse as well!' I bemoan as I muse on how green we still are at travelling abroad, and how clueless I am about what a tourist needs to do with valuables.

'I don't know how they'll even let us back on the ship now!' I wail.

'Yes they will, darling, you worry too much,' soothes Don.

Indeed, he is right, and they allow us back on the ship. Their system uses a primitive form of face recognition from photos they took when we disembarked. The staff in reception were understanding and told me I wasn't the first and wouldn't be the last passenger to be robbed by pickpockets in the port of Barcelona. Reception issues us new boarding passes, and from there, I call our bank in the UK to stop the credit card. I cheer myself up, hoping our travel insurance will compensate us for the stolen cash.

At dinner that evening I'm still feeling rather bruised by the experience but as sod's law would have it, the people at our dining table talk non-stop about their excellent excursion up the *Hill of Montjuic* and their fantastic tapas lunch included at one of the many Michelin-starred restaurants, rounded off by a display of flamenco dancing. I crumble inside, missing this taste of Spain that I'd hoped for.

I'm sorry Barcelona that I part from you in sad spirits. Maybe one day I will get to enjoy all the gifts you have to offer. I hope so.

52. LISBON, PORTUGAL

Losing the cash dampened the delight of every following port, and Lisbon was our first casualty. Without a euro to our name, we couldn't fully savour the beauty of this exquisite city, especially the enticing aroma of freshly baked pastries and the Bica coffees served in the local cafes.

With no money, we have little choice but to get off the ship and just have a stroll around. There's no point wandering through the shops and added to that, there are cobblestones everywhere, which is a problem for Don in his electric wheelchair.

Visually, the cobblestones are a delightful feature of the city, and we learn they are considered public pieces of art that have been around since the 15th century. So serious is this art form taken there is even a special paving school in Lisbon dedicated to the craft called *Escola dos Calceteiros*, but for a disabled person in a wheelchair they are a nightmare, and Don gets all shaken up like he's inside a cocktail shaker—quite apart from me in my inadequate footwear (do I never learn?). I find the cobblestones difficult to navigate in my kitten-heeled shoes, but the cobbles truly are a work of art and I love them.

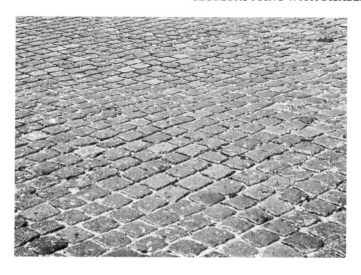

Cobblestones in Lisbon - known as Portuguese Pavements - a beautiful tapestry of artisan skill, but not suited to wheelchairs (or kitten heels!)

So we decide to go for a walk along the estuary where the ground is smooth.

'What's that awful noise?' I observe while strolling towards a large building.

'It's grim isn't it?' Don concurs.

'Sounds like a prehistoric animal in great pain.'

'It's spooky,' chimes in Tim.

Soon, the source of the agonising sound becomes apparent as we walk under the *Ponte 25 de Abril Bridge* (The 25th April Bridge), which is an imitation of the Golden Gate Bridge (in San Francisco), and the reason for the din is clear as we look up.

'Crikey, the traffic is rattling over that bridge on iron! There's no tarmac.'

The dreadful noise spoils this area of Lisbon for quite a distance. On the flip side, Tim, much to his delight, spots a fat squidgy jellyfish in the estuary, though we never did find out what species it was.

As we amble along, we come across a striking, sculptural building adorned with meticulously carved figures etched into its walls. Mesmerised by its beauty, we stop to admire its ingenuity before making our way back to the ship, eager for a refreshing beverage. The piercing cries of the whining bridge, writhing in agony, echo relentlessly, intensifying our gratitude for the tranquillity and serenity that awaits us aboard ship.

One of the most interesting things about Lisbon as a cruise passenger with no cash or credit card is whether the ship will make it under that bridge.

Of course, it does...but if the tide had been VERY high? I join the host of passengers at the front of the ship to watch. It just misses it. It's close. Oooh...

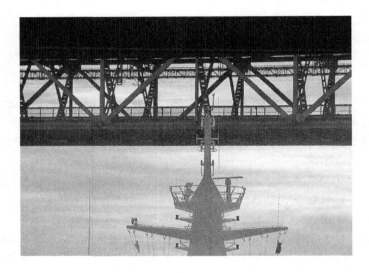

... The ship just misses it...

53. VIGO, SPAIN ~ HOMEWARD BOUND

Our last port of call is Vigo. Once again, our lack of funds spoils our experience in this beautiful port.

Vigo is a fishing town just like Brixham where we live, except that it is well over ten times the size, with some 250,000 inhabitants (compared to Brixham's 16,500).

We can't even buy a lager or try any of the oysters that are seductively displayed in the oyster market. We're completely skint. It's disappointing and I feel rather cheated, but onwards and upwards, there are plenty of things happening on board the ship. Time for a cocktail or two.

The Bay of Biscay is rough on the way home, and Don lies down in the cabin. He feels a tad queasy when he's upright, but I love the bouncy waves and soon find my sea legs as the flat-bottomed cruise ship bobs up and down.

We enjoy watching the ice skating shows on board, though on the return journey, the skaters have a rough time of it and several of them fall over as the ship lurches around. I'd only ever watched ice skating on TV before, and I was awestruck watching the death-defying moves the skaters performed live in front of my very eyes.

Imagine being swung around with your head just inches off the ice, as your legs cling around the neck of your partner who's spinning like a top—and all this on a ship bobbing around on the bouncy Bay of Biscay.

It was tense entertainment.

The sea days can be long but there's plenty to do on board, including sussing out the "Art Auctions" which are a money-spinner for the cruise ship. I go to one of the three auctions hosted by American Art Auctioneers "Park West", lured there because every passenger who attends an auction is given a free print. I'm pleasantly surprised with mine. It's a small but delightful portrait by a contemporary artist, Emile Ballet, of his work *"Interieur"* and I love it[1].

Then there are all the eating places where people can stuff their faces all day if they so wish—from traditional English afternoon tea, to "Sorrento's" where pizza and antipasti are served. I discovered toward the end of the cruise that the food served at these eateries was all included in the price. I'd assumed they'd cost extra. *No wonder there were long queues day and night.*

Despite our missed opportunity, on our last day aboard, we couldn't resist indulging in the exquisite experience of savouring a delightful afternoon tea. As we luxuriated in the fragrant aroma of our Earl Grey, the delicate clinking of porcelain cups resonated all around us. The dainty finger sandwiches, delectable scones, and an array of enticing cakes charmed our eyes and tastebuds. Then, later that evening, we relished the vibrant flavours and tantalising aromas of the antipasti. Even though we had missed out, this last day brought us a moment of culinary bliss.

We're surprised there are cultural events on board. There's a Shabbat meal laid on by the ship for the Jewish community, and although we aren't Jewish, we tag along to experience this occasion and sample the food. We have several Jewish friends in Torbay and we always enjoy their culture when they invite us to join them. The cruise line, of course, knows there will be members of the Jewish community aboard, and so they provide prayer books, kippahs, and dainty lacy head coverings for the ladies.

The cruise ship culture has been an eye-opener for us, and we're not used to being waited on hand and foot like we're the lords and ladies of the manor. It feels odd.

One of the best things about the cruise was meeting some of the wonderful staff, and their hard work and cheerfulness bowled us over. They're always smiling and nothing is too much trouble.

We developed a good relationship with our room attendant, Aniceto, who is from the Philippines. Aniceto has two daughters back home. He finds it hard being at sea for 10 months of the year, he tells us, as he misses them growing up. He continues to delight us each night with his creative towel art as part of the nightly turndown service. When we return to our room after dinner, there it is, another delightful creation, complete with after-dinner chocolates to accompany the artistry. *Where did he learn to do that?*

The chefs also are very artistic with their ice carvings and intricate carvings of enormous melons. The industriousness and hard work of the chefs and waiting staff at mealtimes was in stark contrast to the shoddy food and service we often came across in some UK restaurants.

We are glad to pay our "gratuities" (formal "tips"), which we present to them as cash in an envelope, to show our appreciation. The ship advises passengers of the recommended amount to give each member of staff (room attendant, head waiter, wine waiter, and our restaurant waiters). Fortunately, before setting sail, I had filled the envelopes with the recommended amount of dollars (everything is in dollars on the ship) before being robbed.

All the staff become like a second family to us, yet at all times they remain highly professional.

We can't help feeling it would be better if the cruise line paid their staff a better rate of pay rather than relying on the passengers to supplement their wages with obligatory "tips".

We also found out that many cruise ships are registered in

Hamilton, Bermuda. This also allows weddings to take place on board, though we can't help suspecting that it might also be an accepted tax avoidance loophole, but what do we know?

◆ ◆ ◆

How many eggs does a cruise liner need for a 10-night cruise?

How many gallons of fresh water does a cruise liner produce by desalination in 24 hours?

How many meals are prepared aboard on a 10-night cruise?

How much does it cost to build a cruise ship?

These are just a few of the questions which intrigue me, and so after the cruise, I discover some more interesting facts about our journey and the ship. I've always been interested in nautical things and fascinated by large vessels, partly because I can't understand how all that displacement works, and so for any fellow cruise ship aficionados reading this, here they are:

We sailed over 3500 miles

Flag: Bahamian

Year built: 2007/2008 (in Aker Finnyards Turku Shipyard, Finland)

Maiden Voyage: 2 May 2008

Gross Tonnage: 154,407

Length (overall): 338.9 metres

Crew: 1400 from 65 countries!

Total capacity: 5728 persons

Total cost: $900,000,000

Technical details:

GENERATORS: Six Wärtsilä Diesel 12V46 generators producing 12,600 kilowatts each for a total of 75,000 kilowatts or 103, 345 BHP

DESALINATION: Two Alfa Laval Desalt Steam Flash and Energy Recovery Evaporators
Two Sea-Water Desalination Unit (Reverse Osmosis)

OSMOTEC
233,000 gallons fresh water produced per 24 hour period!
Ice cube production - 65,000lbs per 24 hour period

FOOD AND BEVERAGE
Weekly food preparation - 105,000 meals (including crew)
10 galleys

AVERAGE FOOD CONSUMPTION PER WEEK -
Eggs - 86,400
Slices of Pizza - 18,000
Steaks - 69,000
Individual Yoghurts - 4200
Potatoes - 18,000lbs

Total of 1817 en-suite Staterooms (with 32 of these wheelchair accessible).

The ship has a magnificent bridge, and it is my favourite feature of this fine vessel. I love it.

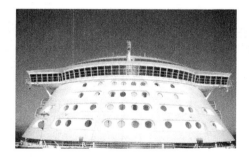

*The magnificent Bridge of Royal Caribbean's
cruise liner Independence of the Seas*

Although there were aspects of cruising which were a culture shock, we enjoyed the experience and thought that not only was it excellent value for money, but that cruising was a good way for us to see a bit more of the world with Don and his no-fly status.

Mind you, I couldn't help feeling that despite all the sumptuous opulence of the ship, a walk barefoot along the shore at my local beach in Broadsands was incomparable.

Despite my purse being stolen in Barcelona[2], we have fond memories of being together as a family in a relaxed manner (unlike driving long distances, shopping for food, preparing our own meals, or searching for places to eat).

I couldn't wait to get back home to see our Sammy-dog. He was aloof with me when I collected him from Elif and he ignored me all day.

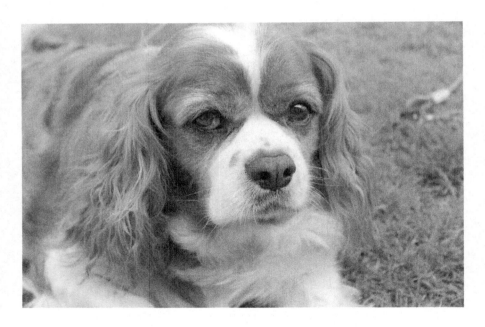

Sammy, totally pigged off with me

[1] I framed the print where it is hanging on my wall as I type.

[2] Our insurance company refunded the loss of 200 euros.

PART SIX - CARIBBEAN CRUISE 2011

54. THE WANDERLUST RETURNS

'I fancy another cruise, darling, what do you think?' muses Don as he flicks through the photos of our Mediterranean sea-fest in 2008. 'They're really fantastic value for money. They work out about a hundred pounds per person per day for full board, all-you-can-eat, with all the entertainment thrown in, and we get to see different places without the stress of driving. We'd never find an accessible hotel in the UK at that price.'

'It'd be lovely to have another cruise,' I concur, 'but if only you'd fly we'd get an even better deal than that, and we could cruise to somewhere more exotic like the Caribbean,' I quip.

'Well, I'm sure there are cruises to the Caribbean from Southampton. I'll have a look online and see what I can find.'

'Good luck with that. I can't see any cruise liner going that far from Southampton!'

In January 2010, my sister and her family had gone on a cruise to the Caribbean for two weeks. It was a fly cruise, however, so Don would be out on his ear on that one.

But on the subject of ears, my ageing father, who lived with my sister in Birmingham, came to stay with us in Brixham while she went cruising. He had a severe hearing disability and had forgotten to bring his hearing aids with him. This led to one of those conversations that is indelibly stuck in my mind. It happened like this: I walked into his bedroom one afternoon after he'd had a nap, and a wall of stifling heat hit me. My father felt the cold, so I'd turned up the heating in his room.

'Are you too hot, Dad?' I enquire.

'Eh?'

'Are - you - too - hot?' I enunciate, a tad louder.

'What?'

'ARE - YOU - TOO - HOT?' I raise my voice a notch more.

'Who?'

'You!'

'Me?'

'Yes, you,' I confirm.

'What?'

'Are YOU too HOT?' I speak with emphasis so he gets the meaning.

'When?'

'Well, now!'

'What?'

'Are YOU too HOT?' I reiterate.

'Are you?' he asks.

'Oh, it doesn't matter,' I say, rolling my eyes, resigned that the conversation must end.

'Eh?'

All I'd wanted was a yes or a no, but I got a who, what, where, and when. Such is life when ears do not work properly.

My father died later that year in August 2010 and although he owned no property (being of a generation that disliked debt of any kind), he'd worked all his life on the track at Landrover in Solihull and had saved some money during his retirement which he left to me and my sister. This gave me a small lump sum, and my wanderlust to travel returned.

'Why won't you fly?' I cross-examine Don as he surfs the net for cruises from Southampton to the Caribbean. 'You can get some great fly-cruise deals, just like my sister did.'

'You saw how I was up the Eiffel Tower. I'd be like that on a plane.'

'No, you wouldn't. It's not like that on a plane. It's just like being on a bus, you don't get vertigo in an aircraft.'

'Well, it's not so much fear of flying, but fear of crashing. We don't even have parachutes. I'm not doing it.'

'But you don't have any fear of crashing an armchair-ski, or your hand cycle, or a dinghy. You almost collided with the wharf in the Hansa dinghy the last time you went sailing with Dart Sailability.'

'That's different.'

Our curiosity about the Caribbean has been piqued, and Don perseveres with his online search, discovering that the *Queen Mary 2* will sail there from Southampton in December 2011. Tim is now 16 and won't want his ageing parents tagging along with him on holidays for much longer, so this will be the holiday of a lifetime for us as a family.

Don rings up the cruise agent and is told that there are only a few places left. The cheapest cabin is going to cost £6000 for the three of us—an inside cabin, £2000 each for a 29-night cruise. Tim has left school and is now at college and the dates fit in well with his term times.

It's a huge chunk out of my small inheritance, but I put my thumb up to Don, who's still on the phone. The agent needs an answer straight away to secure the cabin.

It's excellent value at just over £72 a day each. So we go for it. We'll be sailing to the Caribbean! …via New York! Even better.

There's just one minor snag, though.

55. QUEEN MARY 2

Don will have to use his folding manual wheelchair. He won't be able to take his electric one because it is too wide and won't fit through the cabin door.

This is a blow to us, but it's either that or we lose the booking. All the accessible cabins have gone (so we are told). Don will have to wheel himself up to the cabin, then hobble inside using his arm crutches, and I'll have to fold up his manual wheelchair afterwards. It's not ideal and I'm surprised Don is up for it, but he's triumphant at finding a no-fly cruise to the Caribbean and has set his face towards the challenge. We decide we'll manage somehow. So we pay the deposit and I go up into the loft to see if I can find his arm crutches.

The other snag is what to do with Sammy, our drop-dead gorgeous Cavalier King Charles Spaniel. I had no problem arranging for him to be looked after for a week or two—but a whole month? I decide I'll be able to work something out with all the people who are absolutely in love with him.

We are to set sail on 12th December 2011. I can't wait.

As a young man, my father spent eight years in the Royal Navy and his tales about life on the high seas are another reason I have developed a fascination and interest in all things nautical, even though I'm clueless about the technicalities. I explore some facts about the *Queen Mary 2.* We will sail with the Cunard line, but I discover it is, in fact, the brand name for the White Star Line - the very same company that owned the fated *Titanic*.

The *Queen Mary 2* is a true ocean-going liner and her bow can cut through vast waves—waves that flat-bottomed cruise ships cannot manage. I also learn that it's recently had a multi-million-pound refit, so it should be top-notch when we board in December.

The *Queen Mary 2* made her first transatlantic crossing in January 2004 and comes in at 151,000 gross registered tonnes, can carry a maximum of 2,600 passengers and 1,250 crew (which is less than half of *Independence of the Seas*).

She's 1,130 feet long with 17 decks, and the annual beef consumption would feed a large city for a year.

The ship's whistles imitate the original *Queen Mary* ship and are audible for a radius of ten miles. I will look forward to hearing those.

The day arrives for us to set sail. We do not get free parking this time at Southampton, so we have to travel there by train. We pay for a special taxi that will accommodate Don's manual wheelchair to take us from our home in Brixham to Paignton Station. (Stupidly, there is no railway station in Brixham because the short-sighted Dr Beeching closed it in 1963 along with thousands of other railway stations across the UK. *The mean rotter!*)

Our taxi driver arrives to pick us up and by the look on his face, he's not amused by the amount of luggage he has to load up. We have three large suitcases on wheels, three large overnight bags, two backpacks, a bag with my shoes in, Don's arm crutches, plus two carrier bags with food in for the train journey. Oh, and Don's laptop bag. The driver just about gets it all in his vehicle.

At Paignton station, I push Don in his wheelchair while he pushes a suitcase on wheels with a pile of bags on his knees. Tim acts as porter, pushing and pulling all our other luggage. Don has booked "assistance" at the railway station and the designated guard puts a ramp onto the train and pushes him up into the special wheelchair space. I'm shattered before we even begin the journey.

'How many changes of train have we got before we get to Southampton Central?' I enquire of Don.

'Two. One at Newton Abbot and one at Reading.'

'Oh crikey! You mean to tell me we've got to do this all again, twice?' I quip with sigh. Just the mere thought of getting all our luggage on and off two more trains gives me the heebie-jeebies. 'Wasn't there a train straight through?'

'No, unfortunately. I've booked assistance at them all. You worry too much, darling, we'll get help from the railway staff.'

The journey from Paignton to Southampton Central by the three trains is one of the most excruciating, exhausting, and embarrassing rail journeys I've ever done. How we get away with not paying excess baggage, I'll never know.

At Southampton Central, our struggle isn't over because we then have to get to the port which is nearly two miles away, and it is another grumpy taxi driver who has to load us all into his disabled access car, but he can't refuse us or he might risk losing his license. The thought that we've got to do it all again on the homeward journey gives me the collywobbles, and I try not to think about it. Thankfully, Tim takes it all in his stride, laid-back lad that he is.

At the port, I'm glad when the ship's porters take our luggage from us. We're ushered through the disabled channel to check in and I give our credit card details before boarding the ship.

Now to find our cabin. It's quite a trek to it, and our pile of luggage is neatly lined up along the corridor waiting for us. I open the door, and my heart sinks.

56. NO ROOM TO SWING A CAT.....

Our cabin - Number 6098[1] - is completely unsuitable for a disabled person. It's so small that I literally cannot 'swing a cat' around in it (as the naval saying goes - though the reference there is to the "cat-o'-nine-tails" whip used for flogging recalcitrant sailors rather than a literal cat. I just know these things you see, having learnt about a few nautical bits and bobs).

'It's a bit small,' observes Don, stating the obvious, as he struggles in on his arm crutches.

'And dark. Let's get some more soft lighting on and try to make it more cosy.'

I take a peek in the bathroom. It's the tiniest bathroom I've ever seen in all my born days, with only enough room for one person to squeeze in. There's no way Don will be able to use it at all.

'What's that door there?' observes Tim as he spots a door on the right.

'Maybe there's a room through it to a proper cabin?' contemplates Don as he sits on his bed, trying not to hit his head on the bunk above.

Tim eagerly tries the handle.

But it's locked.

'I bet there's a luxury stateroom with a sea view balcony on the other side, and this is some kind of kids room,' I say, realising what the situation is. 'They've put us in an annexe for children and made a bit of extra money out of it!'

'Well, it's only for sleeping in. We've got the entire ship we can spend our days in,' says Don, ever the optimist.

Resigned to our fate, I get all our luggage into the cabin and start putting away all our stuff—but it's a tight fit. I squeeze the suitcases under the two bunk beds with all our clothes still in them as there's nowhere else to put the garments, and the small wardrobe just about holds all my dresses. *Talk about "living out of a suitcase".*

We make no complaint or demand another cabin, however, even though our hearts are in our boots at having to struggle in a room that is inappropriate for three adults, let alone a wheelchair user.

At sixteen, and over six feet tall, Tim is hardly a child. The cruise agent had been less than honest about the cabin, but if the ship is fully booked, then there is nowhere else for us to go. Furthermore, we are aware that our daily cost is just £72 per person. This is exceptional value, considering the luxuriousness of the ship and the incredible food we will be enjoying. And let's not forget about the amazing destinations we'll be exploring on the other side of the world. This knowledge stops us from kicking up a stink. Besides, the bottle of bubbly and two Champagne flutes[2] on the tiny side table help to take the edge off our disappointment.

We will cope.

We set off to explore some of the ship, which is bedecked with many beautifully decorated Christmas trees, then head for the restaurant to quench our thirst, but I'm at a loss when I see that there are long queues for a glass of juice.

What is this?

The drinks are being dispensed by waitresses wearing vinyl gloves.

'I hope it's not like this for the whole of the cruise!' I moan to Don and Tim as we shuffle along bit by bit in the queue like school children. A lady in front of me who's a seasoned cruiser overhears my comment and advises me it's all because of the

Norovirus protocol.

'In a few days, as soon as the ship's staff are happy there won't be an outbreak, we'll all be free to help ourselves,' she reassures.

The safety drill is next before the ship moves out of port. Clutching our life jackets, every single passenger on board has to assemble in designated areas and follow the instructions relayed to us by a member of the crew. All very boring. But it has to be done.

The time is approaching when we will set sail.

But there's a problem.

[1] *After another refit, Cabin 6098 now does not exist in its previous form and is different to what it was in 2011.*

[2] *There are only two glasses because, on the Cunard cruise line, it is not permitted for anyone under the age of 18 to consume alcohol on board. Tim was 16 when we made this trip.*

57. STORMY WEATHER

There's a Force 10 storm brewing out in the Atlantic.

Commodore Christopher Rynd and his officers are undecided whether to set sail until the storm abates. In the end, they decide to go for it. After all, the *Queen Mary 2* is an "ocean liner". It's what she's built for with her strong bow, able to cut through colossal waves.

So we set off and soon hit the fizzing sea, and I love it. Up up up she soars; the bulk of the ship beneath my body makes me feel twice my weight with my legs shunted heavily underneath my torso. Then down down down she dips, my legs floating away from under me like walking on air.

It's exhilarating. What an incredible feeling.

And that night in my bunk bed, I feel as if I'm being lulled to sleep like a baby in a giant cradle.

Creak creak creak goes her rivets and whatnots as the liner dips down into the 30 and 40-foot waves.

Crash, smash, crash goes the crockery in a storeroom I pass by in the corridor.

And sick sick sick feels Don, poor Don and his funny tummy. So, he really *does* suffer from seasickness after all. He feels nauseous unless he's lying down on his bunk bed. Thankfully, it doesn't affect his appetite, and he eats an enormous meal delivered to our cabin.

In the morning we are still in the thick of the storm, and I get up to make a cup of tea, which I discover is not easy on a ship rolling around. Tim is yet sound asleep in his bunk above me.

He's found some young people his age and had a late night.

It's a struggle for me in the cramped, suffocating shower cubicle, arse stuck up against the clingy shower curtain, trying to soap up. Then, once dried and dressed, a wave of queasiness washes over me. It's most unpleasant.

There's no way Don can even get into the teeny-weeny washroom at all, so I have to assist him with his ablutions—it will be a bed bath every morning for him for an entire month. He'll have to use the disabled toilets on the ship for other things. *Crikey, I hope he doesn't block the toilet again!*

I manage the bed bath, but while I'm trying to get Don dressed, I feel very sick myself and have to lie down, hoping it will pass. *Strange, I was fine yesterday.*

It seems indulging in an early morning cuppa is not a good idea as it sloshes around inside, and we discover drinking on an empty stomach is a major culprit for inducing seasickness.

The ship is still rolling heavily, creaking with every 30-foot wave it dives into. As soon as Don sits up, he feels sick and has to lie down again. There's no way he'll make it to the restaurant for breakfast.

'I'll have my breakfast here in the cabin, darling, but you go and enjoy a proper one served in the posh restaurant,' he encourages selflessly. 'I'll be OK.'

'Are you sure? I must say it's rather grim in here with no windows and being so small.'

'I'll be fine. Just pass me the room service menu and I'll order it over the phone. I'll tell them to bring it into the cabin. I won't be able to get up.'

Oddly enough, even though he feels sick when he's upright, he hasn't lost his appetite one bit and orders an enormous breakfast: fresh fruit, yoghurt, croissant, full English, toast, and coffee. Oh, and the smoothie of the day.

There's nothing else for it. Don has to confine himself to the four walls of the cabin as long as the seas roar. At least the mattress is soft and is to his liking.

Once I've eaten my morning meal, I feel better and find my

sea legs again. I make my way back to the cabin, relishing the physical feeling of the rise and fall of the ship beneath me, and discover Don has eaten the lot and is reading a book.

Tim is still asleep and we allow him to do as he pleases. As his friendships form with other young people on the cruise, he runs on a completely different timetable to us, though we all decide it would be good to eat together for the 'formal' evenings.

Having found my sea legs again, I leave Don and set off to explore this fascinating ship.

My father would love this - especially the storm.

I wind up in the games room and sit watching the 30 and 40-foot waves through a large porthole, and film it using my iPad. An idea comes to me: if I could get Don here to watch the waves, then his nausea will disappear. My logic is that it's like managing motion sickness in a car—if you can see where you're going you feel fine, but if you don't know which way it's turning, that's when the nausea sets in. I show Don the video of the waves and he's up for it. He puts on the anti-sickness wristband he bought, just in case.

We make it to the lift, but he's violently sick *(so much for the anti-sickness wristband).* The Filipino staff are working tirelessly to clean up vomit from passengers who are throwing up all over the ship—I'd seen them at it earlier in the day. They're dressed in fully protective regalia and look like astronauts. And now Don was one of those that needed cleaning up after.

Embarrassed for us both, I seek some attendants to clean up. One of them suggests Don goes down to the Sick Bay to get an injection for the seasickness.

'It works really well,' he assures us.

Don is too ill to go straight away but decides he'll go later. I feel drained and utterly spent by the time we reach the cabin. I make sure Don is comfortable and wash out his soiled clothes, by which time lunch is nearly over. I dash to the restaurant just in time to catch a late meal and I do something I've never done in my life before—I order a large gin and tonic. I'm not a big drinker, but never have I felt the need for a gin and tonic so much as then. It did help to calm me down. *Surely this storm will blow itself out soon?*

After lunch, we make it down to the Sick Bay in the bowels of the ship and spend $60 on the injection, but it has no effect whatsoever and Don is still very ill when upright. So it's back to bed for him. Being horizontal is the only way he can manage his seasickness. But he's very stoic about it and enjoys the room service, having his meals brought to him. His appetite is as big as ever. He eats morning, noon and night, reads books and watches the TV in our tiny room to pass the time away.

Tim finds his sea legs as quickly as me, and he joins in all the stuff laid on for young people.

But on the third night, he disappears.

58. ROUGH SEAS

The storm is still in full swing and at 11 p.m. his bunk bed is empty.

Midnight—no Tim.

1 a.m. Still no Tim. *Where is he?*

I can't sleep.

I try closing my eyes, but I have a fleeting out-of-body experience with every creak and crack of the ship. My mind zooms out from my body, out from our cabin and out from the ship, until my consciousness is hovering far above the raging seas, expanding my awareness of how vulnerable I am on this tiny vessel riding the gargantuan waves, bobbing up and down. Then my mind enters back into my body as quickly as it had left it. I do not feel afraid at all and completely trust the ship and the officers who are in charge of it.

It's nearly 2 a.m. and there's still no sign of Tim. There's no other option but to search for him, and Don is determined to join me. He doesn't feel too bad having eaten a large late-night supper brought to him by room service. All included in the price. *Good-oh!*

We search the decks but it's like a ghost ship at this hour, deserted, with dimmed lights, and a tad spooky.

'Where can he be?' I'm becoming alarmed. 'How can you get lost on a ship?'

'I don't know. I'm really worried now.'

It's past 2.30 a.m. and we're swanning around all the restaurants as we thought perhaps Tim might have been hungry and went for a bite. But they're all closed and in semi-darkness with not a soul to be seen.

We can't look for Tim outside either. The crew has placed hazard tape across all the exits. Due to the storm, passengers are not permitted out on deck; it is forbidden.

'Are you OK?' A crew member wielding a broom stumbles across us.

'We've lost our son. We can't find him anywhere. He wouldn't be able to go outside, would he?' Don enquires.

'Well, it's possible he could have got out, but he'd have likely been swept overboard if he did. It's extremely windy out there,' came the unreassuring reply. *Bloody hell!*

Don and I look at each other, alarmed.

'He wouldn't go out there, would he?' I gasp.

Then, right on cue, we see Tim coming towards us.

Thank God!

He's with a group of teenagers—boys and girls all having fun. They'd been drinking Shirley Temples[1] and playing board games in the Games Room. As they do.

[1] *A non-alcoholic drink made from ginger ale, or lemon and lime soda, with a dash of Grenadine.*

59. SAY CHEEEEESE...

The Commodore's reception party got delayed because of the storm. *Well, it wouldn't do if everyone threw up their champagne all over the Commodore I guess.*

The Commodore's party is a cruising ritual set in stone, it seems. All the passengers dress up to the nines and stand in a line like good little school children waiting to shake hands with the Commodore (or his First Officer depending on which side of the queue you are in) and have a photo taken with him.

Oh wait, but of course!! It's a money-making event, silly me!

The ship must make thousands of dollars from this photoshoot—overpriced snapshots of passengers posing with the Commodore. As I wait in the queue, I wonder what the Commodore truly thinks of this showcase. Does he love it, or does he hate it? Perhaps he's thinking, *'Oh gawd, do I have to shake hands with this blasted lot? I'm sick of this bally gimmick!'*

It must grind him down sometimes, I think.

Despite the still-raging storm, Don is determined to claim his free glass of fizz at this event, so he makes the effort to get up and get dressed. He's not feeling too bad, having eaten yet another huge evening meal brought to him in the cabin. Even Tim gets in on the act and says he'll join us a little later.

We pose with Commodore Christopher Rynd for our obligatory photo with absolutely no intention of paying the $10 for it, but we can't say that in front of him so we have to go through with pretending we want it, and we get our free glass of fizz, and Tim is served a juice. But hawk eyes that Don is, disappointment overcomes him when he spots two elegant elderly ladies next to us, drinking Pina Coladas.

'I'd much rather have one of *those*!' he moans, pointing at their drinks and speaking in a loud voice so that the ladies hear his comment.

'Ah, well, we know the cruising ropes. This is our tenth cruise on board this ship! We get what we want!' is their unhelpful response.

We chat with these delightful live-life-to-the-full ladies and learn that they are both (extremely) wealthy widows. They go on five or six luxury cruises a year with each other.

Now, Don has a unique and Very Special Gift of being able to extract a person's life story in five minutes flat. They tell us all about their late husbands and how they were both left a fortune.

It puts a new spin on the word 'pensioner'.

'We're Agnes and Ethel, by the way, and we're both eighty-seven, you know!'

We clink glasses with them.

'And we're Don and Dawn, and this is our son, Tim. DDT for short, and we're a banned substance, you know!' Don jests (I roll my eyes and inwardly groan, having heard this introduction of us as a family by Don many times before).

On the subject of snapshots, we are harassed by the ship's photographers to have photos taken many times during the cruise. They're there when we get off at the ports, and they're there when we get back on. They come around the tables during lunch and dinner and roam around most events lurking with their oversized cameras. They print off every single photo they take (what a waste!) whether or not you want it. These printed photographs are on display for a limited amount of time in a vast room on the ship, where passengers can look at them. If you don't buy them there and then, they disappear never to be seen again, destroyed.

We bought just one during the whole cruise.

$10.

We thought it was worth at least one shot of us all three together.

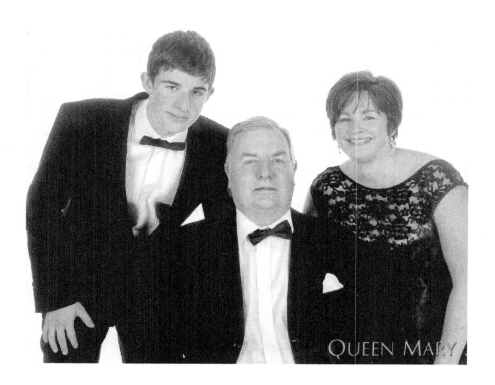

60. UPMARKET

While Don is incarcerated in our cabin and Tim is off doing what teens do with all the activities laid on for them, I try some classes and activities laid on for those passengers who can tolerate the high seas. There are many things to do, but all the ones I fancy often clash.

There's line dancing (not easy to do on a rolling ship!), lectures, the planetarium, and the cinema. No chance of getting bored. Sometimes it all gets a tad overwhelming and I resort to reading a book in the Commodore Lounge or the profoundly pleasant Veuve Clicquot Champagne Bar, minus the champagne, but they don't mind me sipping some water. I discovered that as long as I plonk a glass on the table with something in it, the waiters don't come to take an order from me.

There are also three excellent pianists on board, as well as a fabulous string quartet and a wonderful harpist, so I learn when and where they are playing and enjoy their musical offerings.

The lectures are many and varied. Ted Scull is lecturing on "the city that never sleeps" (aka New York), but that clashes with a dance class I go to.

There are no art auctions like there were on the *Independence of the Seas,* not that I would have taken part. Instead, there is an art gallery by Clarendon Fine Art for wealthy passengers if they wish to invest in top-quality art. Being a nosey parker, I take a look, baulking at the prices. I'm told by one passenger that the lectures have replaced the art auctions.

'I went to hear the Rolf Harris story. It was standing room

only. He's one of my favourite entertainers, such a talented man,' she says.

Oh. Hmm.[1]

[1] *Just over three years later, Rolf Harris was imprisoned.*

61. THE STORM ABATES

On the fifth day, the storm is over, and we are allowed out onto the decks.

It feels like being let out of prison, albeit a very posh prison. The Commodore and his officers had manned the bridge with extra vigilance during the storm and reports from the bridge were of winds up to 70 knots at gale force 11 at times. Commodore Rynd also reported that the ship had "performed exactly as she was designed to do. No other ship could deal with the conditions experienced in such a way."

The yellow and black hazard-stripe sticky tape across the exits comes off, and it's like a new era on board. We discover that the *Queen Mary 2* has a marvellous promenade deck where you can walk around the entire ship.

Just before 11 a.m., we set off outdoors to get a blast of fresh air, all wrapped up in our coats as it's nippy. We're surprised how much we've missed going outside—being cooped up for four whole days has affected us more than we realised. Don is pushing himself in his manual wheelchair on the smooth deck. A nice bit of exercise for him after lying in bed, but before we go twenty yards, Don - as is his wont - strikes up a chat with a couple who are peering over the side.

I carry on, breathing in the crisp air.

Then I hear a dog bark.

That's absurd.

'WOOF!!'

I hear it again.

Do my ears deceive me?

Am I going mad?

Am I imagining things after being cooped up for almost a week?

A dog barking in the middle of the Atlantic Ocean is impossible.

I carry on around the deck and come to a part that's been cordoned off. I can hardly believe my eyes.

62. SEA DOGS

I'm astonished to see several dogs trotting up and down that part of the deck.

So I DID hear a dog bark. Thank goodness for that!

The pooches, brought up onto the deck by the crew responsible for them, are taking their morning constitutional after four days of being cooped up. I think again of our dear Sammy back home, our sweet Cavalier King Charles Spaniel. I've arranged for him to be looked after by three different people over the month we're away.

I'm amazed to learn that some passengers are transporting their pets to New York. Our Sammy would never cope with anything like that, and he'd bark and bark and bark. He suffers terribly from separation anxiety—not just separation from me, but from any human company.

I must show these dogs to Don, so I seek him out and I find him still nattering to the couple he'd met.

'Hey Don, there are dogs on board the ship. Come and see!'

We all make our way to view the canine spectacle. The ever-willing, hard-working Filippino staff are scooping up the dog poop for England as the dogs do their business thick and fast.

Crikey, if it's not vomit they're cleaning up, it's dog shit.

It gave a new meaning to the term 'poop deck'.

There are poop crates available for the dogs - like giant cat litter trays - but they prefer pooping on the deck. Well, I mean they would, wouldn't they? It's reported there are cats and other animals on board too, though we never saw those. Who knew?

I can only imagine what those poor animals went through

during the four-day Force 10 storm. Poor things! They're quite a bunch.

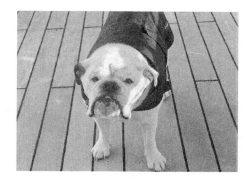

One of the dogs on board QM2
I wonder what the owner looked like?

Then, to my surprise, I'm standing right next to the Commodore himself. He's looking in on the pooches, taking an interest in their welfare. His genuine concern for the animals is heartwarming. What a lovely man.

Here we are together, and I don't even have to pay a cent for it. I get a free photo with the Commodore.

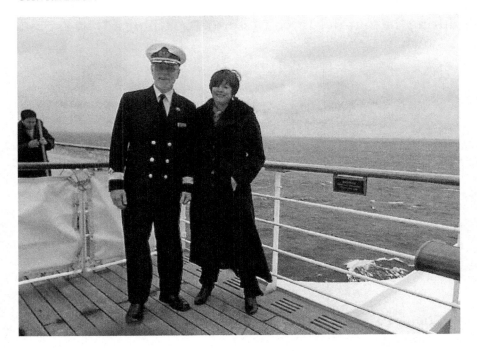

*Commodore Christopher Rynd looks in on the dogs.
Don takes a snapshot just as one of the Filipino
dog wardens is sweeping something up.*

It never even occurred to us that there would be passengers undertaking a transatlantic crossing with their pets. Many passengers would be getting off in New York and a new batch would come aboard for the two-week winter holiday cruise down to the Caribbean.

Don learns from one passenger that a week's cruise from the UK to New York on the *Queen Mary 2* across the Atlantic is now THE way to travel transatlantic to the Big Apple—with or without pets. It's much preferable to a flight, particularly if you fly back, in which case it's also much cheaper because the passenger doesn't have to pay the large airport tax to the British government. Win-win. *Well, it is if you fly, Don!*

63. NEW YORK, NEW YORK!

New York is looming.

After six days at sea, everyone is hankering for dry land. It's a strange feeling being on the ocean waves for almost a week. On the sixth morning, it's bitterly cold but bright and sunny. We're all up at stupid-o'clock to watch the Statue of Liberty come into view. I do not know why, as it's not that spectacular. But it *is* historic, and I tried to imagine myself as a refugee fleeing terror and seeing the statue through their eyes. To them, the statue symbolised freedom and hope.

For some reason, Don and I are not in tune with each other when we get off the ship, and we're very out of sorts. We both have a bit of a tantrum. For me, it's something to do with the fact we're traipsing around the busy bustling streets of New York, yet not going anywhere in particular. Don is enjoying it, but I'm browned off about it. We decide to head for Times Square - somewhere Tim particularly wanted to go and on the way there I see a huge word right in the middle of the street:

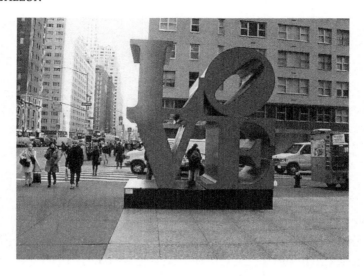

A street in New York - December 2011

I decide I'm whinging about nothing and need to put a sock in it.

Tim pushes Don everywhere in his wheelchair, as I find it rather hard going. In the end, we achieve a fair bit, including plodding through Central Park, which smells like elephant poo; we sing carols with a Salvation Army trio who are out with their tambourines in the freezing temperatures; we investigate Central Station and I'm especially taken with the jazzy ladies' toilets which make the eyes go all funny.

We experience a ride in a specially adapted New York Yellow Cab; we watch the skaters in an outdoor rink; I make it to Macy's and buy a tiny plastic handbag; we get to Starbucks and purchase a special New York mug. As you do. So we find a level and make the best of it in the end, culminating in a visit to the top of the Rockefeller Center. *Who doesn't when they visit New York?* By now, Don's vertigo has subsided somewhat, and he tolerates the height. I'm amazed that he doesn't get dizzy or queasy, but he's fine.

We've done New York. The city that never sleeps. Tick. Next stop: warmer climes with sun, sea and sand in the Caribbean.

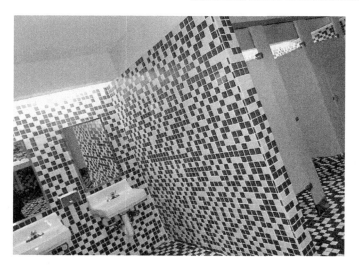

Women's toilets, Central Station

64. CHRISTMAS CAPERS AND DISPOSABLE INCOME

First, however, we have a few more days at sea. We have to sail some 1400 nautical miles from New York to our first port of call in the Caribbean.

Don enjoys playing badminton or shuffleboard on the ship, albeit in his wheelchair. Tim's off drinking Shirley Temples and socialising with his shipmates. I'm not sporty at all, so we all go our separate ways now and again.

Lectures about diamonds are being given as we approach the Caribbean ports that sell precious stones. I toddle along to one, but I'm totally out of my depth. Selling diamonds is a good way for the ship and ports to make extra money out of wealthy passengers, and I'm not one of them.

I go to the cinema instead, and on my way there I walk into the luxurious glazed elevator, where I meet Agnes - the wealthy widow we'd met at the Captain's reception party - standing opposite me looking grey and shaken.

Is she having a heart attack?

'Are you OK?' I ask Agnes, noticing that her back and head are pressed against the elevator wall, her eyes staring unblinking, straight ahead as if she's about to collapse.

'It's terrible!' she says in distress. 'Absolutely awful!' she clutches her chest.

Oh gawd, she IS having a heart attack.

'What's wrong?'

'I've just watched a film at the cinema. Don't watch it, it's dreadful! There's scratching and biting, and sex and... oh, it's horrible!' she laments.

'What was it called? I'm just on my way to watch an opera movie called Carmen.'

'It's called the Black Swan. I thought it'd be a nice film about Swan Lake with ballet and dancing, but it's about killing and blood, it's just ghastly...' her voice trails off as she gets out of the lift, still clutching her chest, looking pale.

Watching Carmen isn't much of a better experience. It's a semi-pornographic production of the opera, with violence. I get up and walk out halfway through. With one thing and another from the previous stormy week, I'm just not in the mood for it.

That evening, as the ship leaves New York with a new influx of passengers for its cruise around the Caribbean, we are put on a different dining table. We're always on the First Sitting at 6 p.m.

I wonder who will join us?

As we're looking at the menu, a mobility scooter whizzes up alongside us.

'I say, I like your snazzy red scooter,' says Don to the elderly lady who parked it at our table. 'Does it go through a standard cabin door?'

'Yes it does, I've hired it especially for the cruise. It's wonderful,' she enthuses. 'I picked it up at Southampton and I'll drop it back there at the end,' she says as she gets off and slips onto a seat next to Don. A young teenage girl follows and sits beside her.

'How interesting. I think I should have done something like that. I've had to manage with my manual wheelchair and it's hard going, especially on these thick carpets.'

We introduce ourselves and Don does his usual "We're a banned substance, you know!" joke.

'I'm Brenda. I'm ninety, you know! And this is young Chloe, she's thirteen.'

'Your granddaughter?' asks Don.

'No! She's my neighbour's daughter. This is her first cruise, and she's keeping me company,' explains Brenda.

Then Don, in his inimitable way, extracts Brenda's life story from her and she tells us she has no children and was recently widowed, inheriting a fortune from her late husband. She has paid for Chloe's cruise.

'I thought my cruising days were over when I lost my husband last year,' she turns to Chloe and smiles, 'but Chloe agreed to come with me, all expenses paid. A good arrangement!'

'Well, you look lovely Chloe,' I compliment her. She truly looks the part in a sparkly evening dress with a flower in her hair, complete with a small matching evening bag and dainty shoes.

'I've bought her several outfits for the cruise. Doesn't she look grown up?' remarks Brenda. 'I've got a wonderful stateroom, and Chloe has an annexe room right next door to mine. They gave me a free upgrade! I'm very pleased.'

A free upgrade?

My heart sinks. *Yes, I know all about those stateroom annexes, unfortunately.*

I feel disheartened, but I say nothing to Brenda about our grim annexe. *Maybe we should have complained after all.*

Chloe is a shy girl, and not very talkative, and I don't quite know how to relate to her, but we have a giggle at Don, who sometimes acts the fool. Tim is nearer her age, but he rarely dines with us, preferring to eat with his mates at the fabulous burger bar.

We spend a pleasant evening with Brenda and Chloe, and like all of us, Chloe is enthralled with the dining experience. Don and I relish all the different courses on offer. There's a soup course, a salad course, a fish course, a main course, a dessert course, cheese and biscuits, followed by tea or coffee and after dinner mints. I have the lot, and Chloe copies me joining in the gourmet affair—she didn't realise you could have all seven courses.

My favourite main dish is the Lobster Thermidor, and my best-loved dessert of all is the light, fluffy, zingy lemon soufflés, which are delectable. When the chefs are paraded into the restaurant for their round of applause (another cruise ritual), I gratefully extend my hearty thanks to them for their culinary skills. They really pull out all the stops night after night, going above and beyond. And it's not just the chefs that are amazing, but the waiting staff are too, laying the tables and serving the guests all the different courses within a two-and-a-half-hour window.

Not only that, the chefs and waiting staff have to do it all TWICE every evening—once for the first sitting at 6 p.m. and then again for the second sitting at 8.30 p.m.

They must be shattered at the end. *How do they do it?*

We like our new dining buddies very much and find it fascinating that Brenda can now spend her husband's fortune cruising several times a year with her young companion. Splendid!

65. TORTOLA, CHRISTMAS EVE 2011

It's warm.

It's balmy.

It's our first port of call in the Caribbean.

We get off the ship, basking in the glorious heat, and head straight for an ice-cold drink before we explore the island. We find a bar and sit outside under an umbrella. I order a Pina Colada and Don orders a lager and lime.

The waiter places our drinks down on the table before us. Don looks at his, purses his lips, and frowns. Don's mind can become befuddled at times, especially when something unexpected turns up such as a bottle of Carib lager with a small wedge of lime in the top. This is not what he is expecting. You see, in the UK, a lager and lime is a pint of lager with a good shot of lime cordial in it. Not to be defeated, he picks up the bottle, puts his thumb over the wedge of lime and shakes it vigorously. It's not difficult to imagine the scene when he takes his thumb off the top. There's a spectacular spray of lager —much to the amusement of the other customers who enjoy this display of total unthinkingness. The spectacle has also been witnessed by the observant waiter, who miraculously reappears with a smile and another bottle of lager (complete with wedge of lime) free of charge. How kind.

'Why did you do that?' I interrogate Don.

'I wanted to taste the lime.'

I shake my head in disbelief.

'Well, you're supposed to drink the lager through the wedge

of lime you daft apeth, not shake it up!'

As we enjoy our drinks, Don gets out his notes about the island. He had done a bit of research at home and printed off some information. We're determined to make the most of this cruise and are trying to resist "just going to the beach" at every port. Tim has wandered off with his mates, so Don and I are at a loose end.

'So what's of interest on this island, then?' I enquire, sucking a piece of pineapple, woefully aware that I should have read up about the islands myself beforehand, but I'd been concerned about travel insurance, passports, tickets and other bits and bobs, quite apart from the pre-holiday pandemonium of packing, sorting out Sammy-dog, watering all the plants and other domestic chores.

'Well, the big thing on this island is reef and wreck diving.' Don looks up at me and I nearly snort my Pina Colada.

The very thought of the pair of us kitted out in wet suits and diving gear is incongruous. Don gets the joke and joins in my mirth.

'There's no way I'd even try to squeeze you into a wet suit,' I tell Don. 'And you'd never manage walking in a pair of flippers, let alone flip backwards over the edge of a boat! Anyway, I'm too much of a coward to even try such an extreme sport. I mean, Brixham is supposed to be a diver's paradise, but it's not our thing at all.'

'Well, there's a zip wire thingy, but there's no way I'm doing that.'

'No, your vertigo might kick in and you'd throw up. I bet these things are very expensive to do, anyway. Let's just go round the shops.'

So that was that.

We traipse around the shops and go back on board early, where I go for a swim in the pool while it's still quiet.

Diving. I ask you! As if we could do such a thing.

Back on the ship, Don has a lie-down and I join in the singing of carols around the grand staircase as the ship sets sail for our next port. What an enchanting thing to do on Christmas Eve. I'm surprised to find that I feel rather moved. Joining in with so many people who do not know each other from Adam, singing their hearts out as one group, is a fresh experience.

When I get back to the cabin, there's a Christmas card, and a beautifully wrapped gift from Cunard. It's a delightful Wedgwood dish. *Nice touch. At least it's not an ashtray!*

We spend Christmas Day at sea as we head further south to Curaçao.

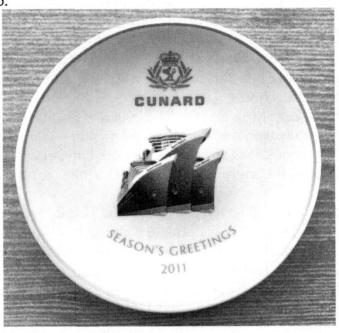

Wedgewood 2011 Cunard gift

66. CURAÇAO

At the beautiful port of Curaçao, many colourful buildings arrest our eyes.

We love it.

We discover just sitting in a local bar enjoying a drink is as nice a thing to do as anything, so we head for a bar where I order one of the local cocktails made with the blue-coloured Curaçao liqueur, and Don orders a lager and lime. I remind Don not to shake it this time.

Feeling invigorated, we eagerly embark on our expedition to discover the wonders of this idyllic island. Vibrant shades of paint gracefully embellish every structure, forming a kaleidoscope of colour that excites our eyes. It's mesmerising, uplifting our spirits with its sheer beauty. While Brixham boasts its own array of colourful buildings, it pales somewhat compared to the breathtaking splendour of Curaçao.

We're surprised to learn that the island belongs to the Netherlands, though the word *curaçao* is Portuguese and it means "*heart*". Over 60 nationalities live on the island.

'Any interesting places to visit here, or shall we just head to the shops again?' I enquire.

Don flicks through the information he has printed off as I push him in his wheelchair.

'There's a museum about the history of slavery on the island if you fancy that? It was the centre of the Atlantic slave trade for many years.'

'Sounds a bit grim. An important subject, but one to read up about later back home. I think I'd just prefer to enjoy the island outdoors. Are there any outdoor places?'

'It says here the island is a diver's paradise.'

'Not again? Stone the crows! We've got no chance of doing that sort of thing. We'll have to give that one a miss. What about food? Are there any interesting local dishes we ought to try? That's more up our street.'

Don browses through his pages.

'Well, it says here that there's a soup made from local cacti called kadushi.' He looks up at me and grimaces questioningly.

'Cacti? Not sure I fancy that right now on top of my breakfast,' I grimace back at him, shaking my head.

'Me neither. It says it's very nutritious but extremely slimy.'

'Anything else?'

'There's a stew called stoba yo-ana, made from iguanas. I'm not sure I could eat any stew right now.'

'Nor me. It's a bit too early in the day. Let's just go shopping again. I want to buy some duty-free perfume. They say it's cheaper here on the island than it is on the ship, and I want to get some of that blue liqueur to make cocktails at home.'

I'm intrigued by the blue-coloured Curaçao liqueur and learn that it's made from dried orange peels from a bitter Seville orange that was imported to the island from Spain back in the 1500s. The oranges themselves are useless, as they are so bitter, but the unripe peels can have their oil extracted and used as the base for the liqueur.

Why isn't the drink bright orange then?

To my disappointment I discover the blue colour is added to make it more saleable and has nothing to do with the drink itself - it's purely for marketing purposes.

As we saunter around the shops, we spot Tim with his shipmates on the other side of the road just as the heavens open and we experience our first-ever tropical downpour. We shelter in a doorway as the rain descends literally like a grey sheet. It's over in a flash, leaving the pavements steaming.

Enchanted by the island's beauty, we head back to the ship after enjoying another cocktail. It's disheartening that we lack a true understanding of the place and can only catch a fleeting glimpse. We'd need a month on each of these beautiful islands to absorb and savour them in all their glory—and even be brave enough to sample the local tasty foods such as cacti soup and iguana stew. *Maybe one day.*

Next stop: Grenada, the Spice Island.

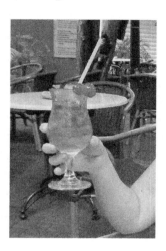

67. GRENADA

As soon as I step off the ship at Grenada, my senses come alive.

The vibrant sound of a steel band fills the air, its rhythmic beats compelling me to move. I can't resist the urge to dance.

Swirling and twirling, I'm joined by another passenger, our bodies gracefully interweaving. I'm oblivious to what others might think and am simply lost in the pleasure of the moment. We happily drop a tip in the collection box, appreciating their talent and contribution to our shared experience.

What will we find at this port? We haven't fully decided, though many passengers have paid to go on exciting excursions on the island.

Excursions are another way that cruise liners make extra money out of the passengers. We read about these interesting tours in the "Daily Digest" sheets given out every night, but they are an extra cost. We accept the choice we make about not booking any, though sometimes over dinner when the other guests enthuse about how marvellous their tour has been, it can be rather deflating.

An excursion at every port would most certainly have enhanced our cruise experience because they ensure passengers sample the essence of the culture - and often the cuisine - of the country. But for those of us who do not pay the extra bucks for these well-organised adventures, we're left at the ports to do our own thing.

Navigating our way at ports isn't always easy and we never know what to expect until we get off the ship. We might be herded like cattle through a myriad of taxi drivers hassling us to go with them, or left to wander around the port shops, or forced to catch a bus into town because the port is so far away from the nearest town.

We are still trying to avoid "just going to the beach" each time and are attempting to get a genuine feel for the culture. We can go to the beach anytime back home in Devon. But we'd read that Grenada has wonderful beaches, so we've come with our swimming gear, just in case, even though we hope we can be a little more adventurous on this island.

'What's of interest here then, Don?'

'There's Leaper's Hill where there was a mass suicide of Kalinago families who jumped over a cliff in the 1600s rather than submit to the French,' Don informs me from his notes.

'Oh, that's grim. I think we'll give that a miss. How horrible.'

'There's an underwater sculpture park where you can go snorkelling.'

I snort a laugh at the image of us snorkelling. *Impossible!*

'Not diving again! Love a duck! They're big on diving in these parts, aren't they? We're out of the game, you and me on that sort of thing. It's way too exotic. We'll have to give that a miss, too. Do they eat iguanas here?'

'I don't think so. Let's see,' Don thumbs through his notes. 'The national dish here is called oil down.'

'It doesn't sound that appetising. What is it?'

'It's a vegetable stew with salted meat. I'm trying to cut down on salt to keep my blood pressure down.'

'I bet it tastes great. I've never tried salted meat—'

'There's a bottomless lake apparently,' Don cuts in before I can persuade him. 'No one's been able to find the bottom of it using sonar.'

'I think we'll give that a miss, too. Let's just go to the beach. We've brought towels, and me and Tim have got our costumes.'

Good job, otherwise we'd be wandering around the shops again.

'Well, we *are* on holiday, and the beach will be relaxing. We can have a snooze in the shade,' Don affirms.

So we get a taxi to the beach and hire some deck chairs. Pushing a wheelchair over soft silky sand is no mean feat, but somehow we manage it.

Included in the price of the deck chair hire is the use of a changing room which is "in the blue building", I'm told by the beach warden. *Great value!*

First, I buy a couple of Pina Coladas. I'm surprised to watch it being made fresh in front of my eyes as the bar attendant juices the pineapple right there and then whereupon she deftly whizzes it into a milky froth. She serves it up in a thin, white plastic beaker which rather spoils the exotic feel of the cocktail. OK, I get it, we're on a beach so no glass allowed, but a white plastic beaker?

It turns out to be the best Pina Colada I've ever tasted. *Nice drink, shame about the cup!*

It's hot in the shade so I long for a swim and seek out the changing room in "the blue building". I wander up and down the beach searching for it, but I can't see a blue building anywhere, so I ask the beach attendant, who points to it a few metres away.

It's not what I'm expecting at all.

68. CARIBBEAN DELIGHTS

The "blue building" (aka the changing room) is a tiny wood and corrugated iron shack, painted a lovely light shade of blue.

I love it.

Inside the changing room, I am intrigued by the resourcefulness of the Caribbean people as I observe the door is held to with a plastic milk bottle filled with sand. *Why bother with a bolt when you can use a milk bottle?*

Perfect!

Despite the poverty on the island, they still take care of the needs of holidaymakers.

Not one to be left out of anything, Don wants a swim too. The tide is coming in and it's not far to the sea, which he shuffles into on his bottom. He's self-conscious of people watching him but determined not to be robbed of swimming in the Caribbean Sea, and it is worth it. The sea is warm, just as Don likes it.

After about half an hour of a gloriously warm water swim, we feel peckish and fancy a bite to eat. So while Don edges himself back to the shore, I get changed in the blue building, and then help Don out of the sea and into his wheelchair. But as the powerful waves draw back, I can see Don is in a spot of bother.

69. GROUNDED

He's grounded like a beached whale and can't move an inch. It's like he's got a lead weight in his pants—he's firmly fixed on his bottom. It's impossible for him to get up into his wheelchair and he's too heavy for me to lift.

He's stuck.

As an enormous wave recedes, I see what the problem is— his swimming pants are full of heavy sand. Don always swims in black elasticated knickers made for very large women, and I must say they look very smart and rather like sporting trunks.

There is nothing for it but to get some help. I can't see Tim anywhere, so I have to rope in some local lads who are very kind and get Don up into his wheelchair and somehow push him back to our deckchairs (no mean feat, as Don weighs 14 stone). I give them all a tip.

With some difficulty, I get Don's knickers off under a towel, as there's no way he'd make it into the blue building. There's wet sand all around his private parts and I do the best I can. I throw the sand-filled knickers away.

Tim turns up just as I'm about to buy a late lunch, and we all try the local chicken dish, which is lip-smacking delicious and attracts the local stray beach dogs. They enjoy the scraps, poor things. They are so sweet and gentle.

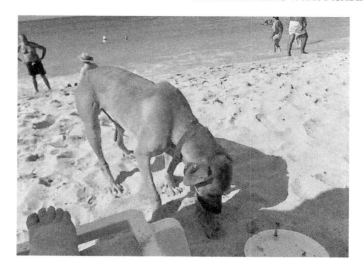

Beach dog eating our scraps

We wash it down with a bottle of Carib lager and enjoy a snooze under the colourful umbrellas.

Despite spending the day on the beach - something we'd been trying to avoid - we decided that we'd experienced more Caribbean culture on the beach than we ever would on an expensive excursion. We loved it.

On our way back to the ship, we wander through a market and I buy some of the famous spices sold to tourists. (Not being an avid cook, they were still in my kitchen cupboard six years later).

Thank you, Grenada, for a fabulous day at the beach.

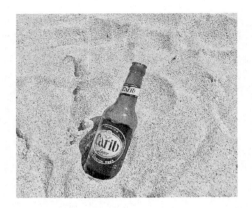

70. CARIBBEAN CHRISTMAS
St Maarten & Barbados

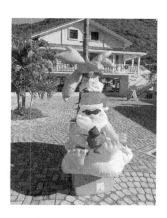

I'm finding spending Christmas in warmer climes a novel experience. What with Santa Claus in sunglasses under a palm tree and a nativity scene in the sun at St Maarten, then witnessing some of the ship's crew enjoying a dip in the warm sea, drinking Carib lager and singing heartily "Walking in a Winter Wonderland!" I'm enraptured by the incongruity of it all.

After our lovely day in Grenada, we submit to spending our time on the beach at the Caribbean ports and embrace the fact that we take joy in the warm sea, being together as a family, and soaking up the local beach life. *Maybe that's what the locals do, anyway.*

In St Maarten, the tide hardly goes in or out and we're

perched right next to it all day. We do not have to move an inch. The tides in South Devon where we live come in and go out many metres, causing everyone to move their beach gear.

Don plays it safe and stays on the shore, but Tim and I enjoy a dip, then quaff a Carib lager while meeting some of the local stray cats.

In Barbados, wondering if we might bump into Cliff Richard (well, you never know), we make our way to Boatyard Beach. The atmosphere is vibrant, amplified by the pulsating beats of loud music filling the air. It's buzzing. The warm sea is crystal-clear and glistens invitingly, just perfect for a delightful swim before heading back to the ship.

But I feel old there. The beach is packed with Bright Young Things—of which I am not one.

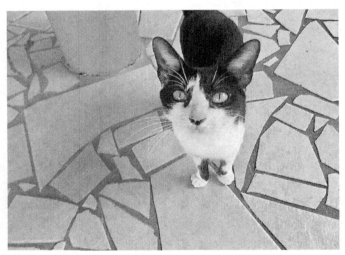

A Carib cat

71. ST. THOMAS

'I'm not sure I'm keen about visiting the island of St. Thomas, darling,' Don remarked one night as we were sipping our Ovaltine a couple of weeks before we went on the cruise. As he prepared for our trip, he meticulously researched each port, printing out information to take with us. However, his excitement dampened when he discovered a cruise ship passenger had been shot to death in St. Thomas.

She was a teenage girl who was caught in crossfire between rival gangs while she travelled in an open-air tour bus in the Coki Beach area. This sort of thing alarms Don. He might have a gung-ho-type attitude about some things, but this story unnerved him.

The shooting had happened just over twelve months previously in July 2010. I'm unsettled by it too, and I can't help projecting the tragedy onto us, particularly as I am prone to catastrophising.

'Well, we could stay on the ship and not get off. The ship will then be deserted and we'll have it all to ourselves, and the pool will be quiet. All the deck chairs will be available,' I suggest.

'It's an idea, yes. We'll see how we feel when we get there, maybe.'

So when we arrive at St. Thomas we're not sure what to do, but in the end, we decide to stick all three of us together, get off the ship and avoid the beaches (since the shooting took place at a beach), but Tim and I take our swimming gear, anyway. Just in case.

We wander off the ship - Tim pushing Don in his wheelchair to give my back a rest - with not a clue where to go. We venture down a road to the right, only to discover that it is deserted, flanked by trees on either side of an unfrequented road.

'I think we should have gone the other way,' I comment, pausing to gaze behind us. 'All the other passengers turned left.'

We find ourselves alone on this desolate road, feeling isolated and exposed. A tendril of fear creeps in as the landscape remains remote, scattered with occasional tin shacks. We have no idea where we are or where we're going. The silence amplifies our confusion, only broken by the faint rustling of wind through the barren trees.

'Yes, I think we should turn around and go the other way,' Don agrees as he takes control of his wheels and does an about-turn. I can see he's beginning to feel panicky, so we all head back towards the dock.

Then we see a man approaching us.

Crikey, what does he want?

His appearance is unhelpful. There's no way to sanitise it. He's rather unkempt, has scabs on his arms and face, has long matted hair and is wearing shabby clothes. As he moves towards us, we do not know whether he is friend or foe.

Will he be hostile towards us?

'Are you lost?' he asks with utmost politeness.

Immediately, his spoken demeanour puts our minds at ease. As the saying goes, looks sure can be deceiving. He's extremely helpful to us, and gentle, relaxed and happy, despite his appearance. He whips out a snazzy mobile phone and calls a taxi to take us to Emerald Beach.

'You'll love it there,' he said. 'Best beach on the island.'

He wasn't wrong—we loved it and had a wonderful time. *Thank you, Lone Stranger in St. Thomas, for your kindness.*

72. ST. LUCIA

Our final port of call before heading back to New York is the island of St. Lucia. The ship wasn't due to visit this island at all, but it had been thrown in at the end because the scheduled trip to Grand Turk had been cancelled due to some problem.

As soon as we get off the ship we're met with an army of taxi drivers touting for business to take us up the mountains. It's all rather chaotic and several drivers offer us different prices.

We are overwhelmed and ignore them as we attempt to reach the exit.

Then we are approached by a driver who boasts of being able to manage Don's wheelchair, which clinches it for us. But when we get to his cab, we discover it's just an ordinary car and Don has to transfer awkwardly into the front seat while the taxi driver wrestles with the wheelchair to fit it into his boot.

The drive up into the mountains is pleasant, but I'm shocked by the poverty on the island.

As we ascend, we see several decrepit, broken-down vehicles scattered along the way. In shady areas, random men are standing on the roadside with half a dozen coconuts at their feet.

I notice many small shacks dotted around which have roofs made from corrugated iron. *Gosh, it must be noisy when it rains!*

And oh! Stupid me, as we drive along roads peppered with banana trees I discover that bananas grow UP. Well, what a revelation that is. I'd have bet my bottom dollar they grew down.

At the summit, we get out to take the obligatory photos where many sellers meet us and show us their wares—

jewellery made from the volcanic rock on the island. I refuse, but one seller is not giving up. He is gentle and respectful, but firm.

'It is our living, Ma'am,' he responds as he holds up an attractive matching necklace and earring set for $20.

I buy the set.

I get it. The local people rely on tourists for their income, and the least I can do is honour that. Considering the quality of the items, $20 was a small amount to pay.

Our taxi driver is friendly and chatty as we head back down to sea level. We decide to round off the day near the beach and town centre. Tim can enjoy a swim while we mooch around the market. We haven't been to a large Caribbean market yet, so we decided to tick that box. The taxi driver assures us he'll be ready and waiting to take us to the ship at 4.30 p.m. prompt. *Can we trust him to keep his word?*

Don and I wander towards the market, but the town is dusty, hot and sticky, and not only that, I've never seen such deep kerbs in all my days. St. Lucia is not geared up for wheelchairs. The cobblestones shake Don up, and after buying a few souvenirs, we return to the beach where our taxi will pick us up. The afternoon is wearing on and we just have time for an ice-cold drink before we get our taxi.

But where is Tim?

73. WALKING IN A WINTER WONDERLAND...

'Tim?! *Tim?!*'

I walk up and down the beach, calling him.

Where on earth is he?

I'm getting distraught as my fragile emotions surface and I start to catastrophise. We both look up and down the seafront.

I become alarmed and irrational.

'What if he's been killed!' I sob as red lights flash in my head, high-alert danger sirens going off in my brain. I'm convinced bandits have abducted him.

We find our taxi driver who, true to his word, is ready and waiting for us half an hour early and he sees the state I'm in. We explain we've lost Tim. In a flash, he's got together a posse of young local lads to help us. They are terrific and extremely kind, trying to calm me down. They ask what Tim is wearing and they send out a search party truly going the extra mile and more.

'Don't worry Ma'am, we'll find him, please don't worry,' assures the leader of the pack.

And find him they do, bless them. Tim had inadvertently wandered off down the farthest end of the beach, unaware that we were in a panic.

'Your parents are looking for you, man! You should see what you've done to your mom!' are the words that greet Tim as he's approached by one of the young men who tracks him down, recognising Tim's T-shirt.

The relief at seeing Tim is overwhelming, but I'm too exhausted to tell him off, and there's no reason to anyway as he'd only been having a good time with his pals.

To my shame, in my distress, I completely omit to give the group of lads a generous tip for their kindness. If only I could rewind the clock.

In the taxi on the way back to the ship, I can't stop crying for some reason, and the tears just keep on flowing along with intermittent, involuntary sobs. Maybe it's the last straw, for, back on board, I know what I will have to face.

74. CORRIDORS

I'll have to do some laundry runs up and down the extremely long corridors to the laundrette on the ship. I do all the laundry myself as it's an added cost to use the ship's laundry service, and I'd rather have a glass of champers with my meal instead.

Cruising for an entire month means I have to do at least one wash a week, though, in reality, it turns out to be two or three loads a week.

The laundrette is located at the opposite end of the ship from our cabin on Deck 6. *Well, it would be, wouldn't it?* It's quite a trek (bearing in mind that the QM 2 is over 2000 ft long).

It involves humping the laundry to the launderette to load the washing (that's if you can find an empty washing machine as everyone else seems to do it at the same time as you), then 45 minutes later going back to take it out and put it in a dryer, then 30 minutes later going back to take it out of the dryer and iron it, then cart it all back to our cabin where I stuff it all into our suitcases under the bunk beds. *At least it's good exercise.*

The chore is a regular bugbear of the cruise and is not something I want to do on holiday, but there is no use having a strop about it. I just have to grin and bear it.

The long corridors are also a challenge for me pushing Don in his manual wheelchair. He helps as much as he can by propelling himself (he's developed a lot of upper body strength because of his disability over the years), but he can't push himself on the thick, plush carpets which makes using a manual wheelchair on board virtually impossible. The twinges in my back are concerning.

Will my back hold out for the whole month?

◆ ◆ ◆

The next day we spend at sea and in the afternoon I do two laundry runs.

By the time I finish, I'm pooped.

I'm hot and bothered, but there's still an hour before "Afternoon Tea" is served. Tim is off somewhere with his young mates and Don is playing badminton in his wheelchair. His competitive streak emerges during the cruise, and he enters any competition he's able to take part in. He often wins, evidenced by a growing collection of certificates and badges in our cabin.

I can't join him in playing badminton because I have no hand-to-eye coordination. Besides, the last time we played it in doubles, I ended up being the shuttlecock-picker-upper. So I decide I'll cool off in the enchanting whirlpool on Deck 11 instead.

Perfect.

I'd seen the whirlpool a few days before when I looked down from Deck 12 and thought how lovely it was—fairly quiet too, with only a handful of people sunning themselves, drinking cocktails. So I get changed, buy my cocktail and set off to experience the delights of the whirlpool, unaware I'll be facing an unforeseen revelation.

75. THIRD CLASS

I can't get through to that part of the ship on Deck 11 at all.

Am I at the wrong end of the ship?

I often get lost aboard ship, confusing the front from the back, but I was sure the pool was aft. Mystified, I go to the opposite end, but that's no good either. I head to the lift area to find a map of the ship and ask a crew member who informs me they only allow certain passengers through to the Deck 11 pool area.

Crikey, I didn't see that coming. Damn!

The *Queen Mary 2* has a class system on board (even though it's not advertised as such, it exists. Well, it does from my perspective, anyhow). The ship reserves certain parts exclusively for passengers who pay tens of thousands of pounds for the luxurious suites, denying access to those in the cheaper cabins.

Fair enough.

I get it.

They need a bit of private space; they've paid thousands of pounds for their suite and they don't want to fight for a deck chair every time they wish to sunbathe. Nevertheless, I was a tad taken aback by it.

In that respect, sailing with Cunard on the *Queen Mary 2* was a different experience to being a passenger with the Royal Caribbean Cruise Line where we were all equal - we all had the same access to all the same places.

I realise the class system which had operated on the Titanic White Star Line is still operating somewhat on the *Queen Mary 2*, albeit in a semi-subterfuge manner. Even the dining areas are separate where the wealthy passengers dine in the "Princess Grill" or the even more salubrious "Queens Grill", which is strictly reserved for passengers travelling "first class". Being a nosey parker, I wondered how their food differed from ours. *Oh well, I'll never find out.*

Instead, I take a swim in the second-class pool and then join Don in the queue for Afternoon Tea, which is held daily in the elegant ballroom. We aren't that hungry, but we can't resist it. Such exquisite morsels lure us.

In the elegant setting, dainty cucumber sandwiches and smoked salmon sandwiches are meticulously served, along with crumbly scones and miniature cakes, adorned with intricate designs. The delightful aroma of speciality teas, including the comforting scent of my beloved Earl Grey, envelops us. Impeccably dressed white-gloved waiters serve each delicacy with utmost grace. The soothing melodies of a string quartet create a harmonious backdrop, enhancing the overall ambience.

Then, after a while, a band plays elegant ballroom dances. "Gracious living" Don calls it. I guess you could call it that, perhaps.

During every Afternoon Tea, a diverse group of passengers, both wealthy and not-so-wealthy, mingle together. We find ourselves in the company of three individuals—a married couple and a widow. As fate would have it, the husband openly discusses his observations of a distinct class system aboard the ship, sharing his unfiltered opinions about it and the upper-class passengers he's encountered, not realising that the widow is one of the "first-class" passengers. A tendril of tension pervades the air as she abruptly rises from her seat and storms off.

Awkward.

We are horrified at the clanger he's dropped, and after a red-faced "Oh dear!" from him, followed by nervous giggles, we concentrate on watching the dancing in silence.

The ballroom dancing at the Afternoon Teas is extremely

popular, and the ship provides professional male "escorts" to dance with single ladies. These escorts are all mature men over 60 with an official badge. They have a good eye for picking out women who want to dance.

The ballroom dancing is also popular with people of all ages and nationalities, and we enjoy watching them dance from the sidelines. The Japanese couples are expert at it, dancing with much elegance and professionalism.

Even Tim and his gang come along occasionally, holding their cups with curled little fingers, experiencing the high life.

As we are getting ready for dinner later that evening, I tell Tim about my observations concerning the "class" system on board.

'Oh I know,' Tim confirms, 'one of the girls in our group, Tilly, is in the most expensive suite on the ship with her family. Her grandfather paid over ten grand for it. They all dine in the Queen's Grill every night.'

Our tiny cabin certainly feels third class and I wonder whether the third class passengers on the *Titanic* had more spacious cabins than the one the cruise agent fobbed us off with. But we still do not make any complaint, and we're grateful to be aboard this magnificent vessel—a truly unique experience for us. Besides, for £72 a day each it is incredible value. How else could I get to see the world in such luxury? Plus, there are many marvellous parts of the ship where we may go, so there's nothing to gripe and grumble, whine and whimper about in reality.

76. SEA DAYS

'Take your flute,' my sister had told me when I informed her we would be cruising on the *Queen Mary 2*. She said that on her cruise to the Caribbean, there'd been karaoke and talent shows. So I duly packed it along with some music.

There's rarely a moment of the waking day when there isn't some activity going on aboard, including cultural and spiritual events, as well as lifestyle classes, which lured passengers with the offer of health advice but were really a ploy to sell "health packages" by the company running the class. I attend only one of these.

We are invited to join a Hanukkah celebration and one of the Shabbat meals provided for the Jewish community on board. Don, in his inimitable way, was chatting with some of them over lunch one day and told them that although we weren't Jewish ourselves, we had several Jewish friends in South Devon. The speciality cuisine laid on by the ship for these cultural events was delicious, especially the potato latkes and the Jewish delicacy of gefilte fish.

We also attend one of the Anglican Christian services led by the Commodore, with hymns, prayers, and Bible readings. This Sunday ritual seems to be a tradition going back many centuries, ingrained in seafaring history. I wonder what happens if the Commodore or his officers are atheists? Maybe they have to pretend? There are also separate services allowed on board for Catholics and free church worshippers.

Much like the *Independence of the Seas*, life aboard is comparable to living in a small city. You can start the day with an early morning Yoga class at 6 a.m. and end with a disco well into the early hours.

But the *Queen Mary 2* is a more intimate cruise liner than *Independence of the Seas*, with almost half the number of passengers and we much prefer the smaller ship. When you are new to cruising, there are aspects which might not always sit well, but it's undeniable that the staff and crew are amazing and work extremely hard. You just long for them to get a decent wage.

What happens if you fall seriously ill on a cruise ship in the middle of the ocean?

A scary thought. It could happen to anyone.

Well, on a sunny afternoon during our cruise across the Caribbean islands, it does happen.

A sense of drama permeates the mood aboard as word gets around that a passenger has had a heart attack, necessitating a medical evacuation. Curiosity sparks within us, drawing us to the deck where we expect the imminent arrival of a helicopter.

The sound of whirring blades cuts through the otherwise tranquil atmosphere, mingling with the murmurs of concern from the onlookers. With our eyes fixed on the sky, we witness the pilot's determination as he attempts multiple times to land on the ship. Suspense rises as the crowd holds its breath, conscious that the clock is ticking for the patient.

Will he be able to land?

Finally, as the helicopter gracefully touches down on the deck, relief washes over us, eliciting a spontaneous round of applause to honour the pilot's unwavering perseverance.

In our "Daily Digest" sheet, we discover that there will be a talent show on New Year's Eve. With several days at sea before we hit New York, we put our names down to take part in this passenger performance-fest and attend the rehearsals.

I'll be playing Bach's *Prelude No. 1 in C*, a simple, but delightfully pretty piano solo.

Then Don and I will play Bach's evocative and poignant *Sicilienne* as a duet, me on the flute accompanied by Don on the piano.

We are the only classical music act and out of kilter with the other offerings, which makes me feel a tad nervous. The show will take place in the enchanting ballroom where there's a superb Steinway grand piano. *Oooh…lovely.*

These talent shows are an enormous amount of work for the staff organising them, especially for the unlucky pianist responsible for sourcing any music needed, accompanying the entrants, and rehearsing all the acts. On this voyage, it's a wonderful young pianist called Adam, and Don discovers that he'd studied Musicology at Birmingham University and had never intended to become a cruise pianist.

I can only imagine the staff must dread these talent shows. We're a motley crew, yet a courageous bunch, putting on a diverse array of performances for those passengers bold enough to attend the show and subject their ears to our amateur musical offerings.

Some singers are excellent, however, and I'm rather envious of them. It was a tremendous disappointment for me to submit to the fact that I'd never be a solo singer. I just didn't have the vocal tackle to be a soloist (though I can hold a line in a four-part choir).

The classical pieces Don and I perform are rather out of kilter with all the modern and popular acts from the other entrants, but I'm pleased with my rendering of Bach's Prelude No.1. The amazing Steinway piano is incredibly responsive and does exactly what I want it to, including an effective gradual crescendo towards the end of the piece as the music builds to a climax and then resolves.

Our duet goes well too, even though I fluff several notes on my flute. But nothing too bad.

Then after we finished, Adam, the pianist responsible for organising the event, accompanies one of the singing acts. It's a rendering of the song "People" but it's sung pitifully out of tune and completely out of time by the participant who's a middle-aged lady of a similar age to myself. The song "People" has a complex melody, and it's difficult for an inexperienced singer to perform and bring it off well. How Adam navigates it is quite astounding as we hardly recognise the tune at all, and as I sit and listen I'm reminded of the celebrated accompanist Gerald Moore when, in a fit of exasperation at the dodgy intonation of a soprano he was accompanying, had said, "Madam, I can play the black notes, and I can play the white notes, but I can't play in-between the cracks."

I have to suppress a giggle.

'Well done Adam,' Don congratulates Adam's pianistic feat at the end of the song.

'Was it OK? I found that really challenging,' Adam responds.

'You worked wonders, not an easy act to accompany.'

After the show, the lady who'd sung the song was blissfully unaware of how bad it was, yet Adam had done a wonderful thing for her.

'I can tick that off my bucket list now!' she exclaimed triumphantly, radiant with a sense of accomplishment and grateful for the opportunity. And indeed, that was the principal aim of the Talent Show, to empower the passengers in their artistic endeavours, whether good or bad. To that end, it achieves its goal.

Many other acts are of a very good standard indeed. There's a variety of offerings with poems, jokes and dances. The audience seems enthralled, expressing their appreciation with polite clapping between each number. The final act is a husband and wife duet rendering of Andrew Lloyd Webber's "All I Ask of You"—it's splendid and raises the roof with rapturous applause and was an excellent choice to conclude the event.

At the end of the show, as Adam passes me by, he makes an

unsolicited comment to me.

'You played well. You'll be joining the staff soon.'

This small but encouraging remark remained with me long after the cruise had finished and helped to change my whole life. Adam had said this, unprompted, without sarcasm, and I believed him. It was a seed sown—a small encouragement for me to go professional one day as a pianist. Thank you, Adam.

Being New Year's Eve, we're all given party poppers and some rather dapper party hats to wear at dinner (no mean feat for the crew to give out over 2000 hats). The night wears on, and the festivities on board are in full swing as the countdown to the new year closes in, with the sound of laughter and music in the air.

But I'm not in the mood for partying.

Instead, we venture out to the stern of the ship on the peaceful promenade deck, seeking solace in the beauty of the starry sky.

It's a balmy night.

Serene.

And a rare opportunity. Because here, out on the ocean, the sky is devoid of the contamination of artificial light. We gaze and gaze at the Milky Way, not wanting the moment to end. A myriad of shimmering crystal-clear constellations stretch out before us: each star a sun, millions of miles away.

As 2011 slips into 2012, for us, time stands still.

I can hardly breathe.

I've never seen such countless twinkling stars in all my days, and they bring a lump to my throat. I love them so much.

We're at sea for two more days before reaching New York, but at dinner on New Year's Day, something is terribly wrong.

77. GENERATION GAP

Brenda and Chloe are late joining us, and we're finishing our starters as they appear. We apologise for starting without them, but it's clear they're both extremely unhappy. Their faces say it all. Chloe looks very upset and is on the verge of tears. Brenda looks like thunder.

They will not sit next to each other and I try to take Chloe under my wing to cheer her up - but how to connect with a tearful thirteen-year-old?

During Don's conversation with Brenda, I attempt to lighten the mood by impersonating our Bulgarian wine waiter, Vasil. He always asks me if I want "more wine?" but his lovely accent elongates the vowels, making it sound like "Moorra waine?"

His slow and seductive inflection ascends in tone as he leans over and pours before I can say "no". Chloe thinks this is hilarious and my imitation of him cheers her up for all but two minutes.

Then, right on cue, Vasil appears,

'Moorra waine?' he says, decanting a top-up with his charming smile. I take a moment to get Chloe's troubles off her mind by asking Vasil if he has any family back home.

'A wife and a son,' he says. 'He is five years old.'

'You must miss them. Do you get a chance to see them often?'

'I haven't been home in five months, but we chat online. It is hard at times.'

Reading between the lines, the issues between Brenda and

Chloe indicate that they've had a disagreement and have fallen out.

We try to lighten the atmosphere and Don gets his usual bout of giggles when the food waiter uses his "crumber" to clear away the crumbs after the starter (Don is a very messy eater). This tiny tool that the waiter whips out to clean the table with amuses Don no end. He loves it. All the waiters are skilled in the fine art of crumbing a table, using a crumber which is a small curved piece of metal. They elegantly clear away crumbs and other small table detritus into a napkin or their free hand, with a flick and flourish of the wrist. But Don accuses the waiter of clearing the crumbs into his lap as he larks around. His humour over this nightly dining drama is infectious and has us all laughing, including the waiter, along with Brenda and Chloe. But the light relief is temporary as the atmosphere brought to the dining table by them becomes even heavier as the evening wears on.

By the end of the cruise, Brenda and Chloe are not on speaking terms at all, and I think it would have come to blows if they hadn't been the ages they were.

It turns out that Chloe had abandoned her benefactress, preferring to go off to the pools on her own and mix with young people her own age, much to the chagrin of Brenda, who'd paid for Chloe's month-long cruise to be her constant companion. But it's all too much for young Chloe, and being a lady's companion is a role even a mature woman would have found challenging. I feel for them both - Brenda's expectations have not been met and have cost her a lot of money, but poor little Chloe is too young and as time wears on, she is flagging with the responsibility of it all.

It's a sad end to what should have been a happy time for them both.

They can't wait to get home and part ways.

Our cruise is coming to an end, and by the final and fourth week - which is six days at sea as we sail from New York back to Southampton - we are hankering for home. I want to see our beautiful Sammy-dog, who has oodles of character. He must be feeling abandoned, and he is in my thoughts constantly.

The last day arrives, and we receive our invoice for what we have spent on several drinks we've had on the cruise, and a few purchases, plus the "gratuities" we must pay. On this ship, gratuities are added to our cruise bill - there's no cash in envelopes this time. The tips are calculated at a daily rate per passenger and will be shared between several members of staff. It's not that we aren't grateful for their hard work and excellent service (always with a smile), but it's a disappointment that the ship doesn't pay them a decent wage and expects us to top up their salaries. I wonder how the staff truly feel about gratuities?

Over the entire month of the cruise for three people, the "gratuities" tot up to a fair amount, and I'm not happy about it. But when I examine the invoice to see what we owe, I'm in shock.

78. IT'S IN THE DETAIL

It's hundreds of dollars more than I'm expecting.

After scrutinising the invoice, it's clear that the culprit is Tim. There's a vast amount owing for "satellite communications" - internet stints from the ship, which are exorbitantly overpriced.

I have to pay the bill. We can't get out of it. Cunard has our credit card details, which we gave before we set sail. It is part of the cruise contract.

We'd told Tim not to use the internet aboard the ship. We never used it either. Somehow it seems odd, and I didn't think Tim would go against our instructions.

'Tim, what's all these internet charges? Look! Here on our invoice!'

He tells me it's not him. He hasn't used the ship's onboard internet facility at all. I believe him and I know he wouldn't lie to me about it. But how can we prove this to the ship?

Tim and I venture down to reception to challenge them over it and put the ball back into the ship's court by asking them to investigate. I'm not feeling hopeful they will believe us and have no idea how we can convince them.

But to their credit, they do investigate it and take our objections seriously. By some quirk of fate, they have (what seems to me at any rate) a brilliant technical guy who soon finds out that there is indeed a problem. He also discovers that we aren't the only ones to have this dilemma - several other families have had the same issue.

It transpires that the real culprit is young Tilly, the thirteen-year-old granddaughter of the richest passenger on the ship who'd dined every night in the Queen's Grill. Despite her grandfather's wealth, she, too, had been banned from using the ship's internet facility. So she'd done it by stealth. It was simple; anyone wanting to use the internet could do so by providing their name, cabin number, and date of birth. The entire group of youths, including Tim, had freely shared this information with her and she'd had an internet-fest every single day and night.

Just goes to show, there's always one. As rich and privileged as she was, she'd used deception to get what she wanted. To my great relief, the ship assures us they will look into it and refund us the money.[1]

It's our last day aboard, so I hope for a good outcome regarding the internet charges and decide to make the most of our final meals. By the time I've waited in the queue at reception and packed a few things in our suitcases, it's lunchtime. Don and I go down to the restaurant and Tim heads for the burger bar.

'They're the best burgers I've ever eaten,' he informs us.

I often wish I'd tried one.

[1] A few weeks after we returned home, Tilly's grandfather, to his credit, paid for the internet fees once the ship could prove to him beyond doubt what had happened, and we got our money back. It must have cost him thousands as there were several families affected by Tilly's misdemeanour. *What on earth did Tilly do on the internet?!*

79. DODGY DINING COMPANIONS

'I don't want to watch some tart kicking a football around a pitch!'

The middle-aged man hogs the lunchtime conversation as we, his captive audience on the table for eight, have to endure an hour and a half of his misogynistic opinions.

'It's obscene these women running around a football field!' he continues as we politely eat our starters.

Women's football is in its infancy, and this passenger has strong views about it. I have the urge to give him a piece of my mind, but I keep quiet. I'm not going to let this arrogant brute spoil my last lunch, so I tune him out. We all hold our tongues as we don't want to embarrass his wife, who's as quiet as a mouse and doesn't speak a word.

We always eat in the restaurant for lunch and dinner, but at lunchtime, we never know whom we'll end up eating with as it's all down to the whim of the head waiter who has to juggle the tables. You have to sit where you're told once the waiter knows what size table you're happy with.

'Table for six or eight,' is always Don's reply, as he loves meeting people and chatting. But if you get trapped with a highly opinionated passenger who gets on their soapbox, it can have its downside. When lunch was over, it was a relief; but I was left feeling angry that I wasn't able to give Mr No-Women's-Football a piece of my mind.

Our final evening dinner with Brenda and Chloe is subdued, and the frosty atmosphere between them hardens. We feel sad for them and try to make the most of it. Tim joins us and he sits next to Chloe and chats to her, which helps.

Finally, it's time to disembark. The journey from Southampton to Paignton by three trains is agonising because of the amount of luggage we have, but yet again, we avoid getting charged for excess baggage.

The first thing I do when we reach home is fetch Sammy, our dog, and he ignores me when I collect him from Barry and Helen, who'd looked after him during the final week.

'Sammy's spent the whole week curled up on Barry's lap,' informs Helen, 'apart from when I walked him. He's such a lovely boy.'

Despite the luxury and opulence of the ship, I still had mixed feelings about the whole cruise experience, and there were aspects of it I found alien, which left me feeling uncomfortable, though it was difficult to explain why.

Since backpacking and camping are not my thing, even if Don could manage it, sailing on a liner does have some advantages. But there's a relentlessness about cruising; a sameness, yet a differentness, all rolled into one. It's certainly got a "culture" to it, and it's a culture I can't quite reconcile myself to. I'd much prefer a different type of holiday, but we have limitations with Don's disability and his no-fly status. We are always only "tourists" and never really get to taste and savour the ports sufficiently. All we get is a fleeting microscopic whiff, and only then the veneer of it laid on for the cruisers.

Having said that, one lingering aura of the Caribbean for me was that they truly valued tourists. Of course, we brought money into their ports, but I sensed it went deeper than that: I noticed they sincerely enjoyed hosting us, giving us the best experience they could, in contrast to some European attitudes where tourists are perceived as a nuisance. The warmth of the

Caribbean people lingers with me to this day. I genuinely felt valued and welcomed as a tourist in the Caribbean, and I will always be grateful for that.

Nevertheless, I was happy to return home. A whole month away was a bit too long. And I was £6000 poorer[1].

In hindsight, would I have done it?

It had been tough as a carer on the cruise and it wasn't the relaxing holiday I'd hoped for—especially with the awful laundry runs. But overall, considering the only way to see more of the world is by ship, we'd had a great time and made some lovely memories together as a family.

The laundry runs faded into the past and were replaced by good recollections of family bonding.

Yes, it was worth it.

We also fell in love with the *Queen Mary 2* ship. There is definitely something special about her, and we had to admit that the standard on board was exceptional. We'd love to sail on her again one day.

And what of Adam's lovely comment about my meagre talent show offering?

Quite simply, it was life-changing.

It encouraged me to contact the National Trust to be a volunteer House Pianist at Greenway House and Coleton Fishacre, not far from where we live. I worked up some of my classical pieces and got used to playing in front of people again with the aim of going professional once I'd mastered my nerves.

Fast forward two years and I get my first gigs as a hotel pianist.

Thank you, Adam!

[1] *Tim gets a full-time job shortly after the cruise and kindly reimburses his fare, which I use as a deposit on a shiny black baby grand piano.*

PART SEVEN - P&O CRUISES

80. MEDITERRANEAN CRUISE - 2015

I move the chicken around on my plate and my heart is in my boots.

It's a tasteless school-dinner-type meal and I'm intensely deflated. So much for the "fine dining" advertised in P&O's brochure.

Don and I (no Tim this time) are on board the *Oriana* for a cruise around the Med. I gaze out of the window at the dock wall in Southampton, which is looking grim on the dark and rainy February evening. Not only is the food disappointing, but we're going nowhere on this first night. There's a problem (though we're not told what it is) and the ship's staying put in port. But fair dos, the company does at least refund some of the fare for every passenger as compensation.

On top of all that, we'd had the most exhausting journey from Brixham earlier that day by train, and to save a bit of money had skipped taking an accessible taxi from Southampton Central Station to where the port was and we walked instead.

It was a big mistake.

The "28-minute walk" (3 minutes in a taxi) to the port turned into a 45-minute hike for us with the enormous amount of luggage we had. It was a struggle.

The only consolation is our lovely spacious, accessible cabin —and we have a porthole! *Yippee!*

It's an "obstructed" porthole mind (obstructed by a lifeboat outside), but it's a porthole nonetheless and it lets in natural light during the day.

We set sail the next day, heading for Gibraltar and things aboard improve dramatically. I needn't have worried about the food. My favourite dish, Lobster Thermidor, is on the menu on the second evening, and I perk up. We enjoy a fancy starter and the Thermidor arrives.

'Oh drat, I've left my blood pressure pill in the cabin,' notes Don.

'I'll fetch it. It'll be quicker for me.'

I dash there, conscious of my food getting cold, then wend my way back into the restaurant. But I'm puzzled to see Don coming towards me. *What else has he forgotten?*

81. DÈJÁ VU

As we draw near to each other, I see that he's been sick all down his dinner jacket and is throwing up his Lobster Thermidor into his napkin.

All the other guests are being very polite by ignoring him as he weaves his way around the dining tables and I about turn and follow him out of the restaurant to our cabin, where I help to clean him up. The gentle rocking of the ship into the choppy Bay of Biscay has triggered his motion sickness. That's the end of the meal for him. He has to lie down.

I learn that the ship has stabilisers to reduce rolling motion by 90%, but it seems they only kick in at a speed of 19 knots, and they weren't of any help at all that evening.

I'm determined not to miss out on my lobster (a rare treat for me), so I head back to the restaurant to finish my meal even though it would be stone cold.

But it has gone. *Bugger.*

Just as I'm about to protest, our lovely waiter brings me a fresh Lobster Thermidor, hot and steaming. I order a large glass of Sauvignon Blanc.

82. OLD ORIANA

After the dodgy start, everything improves on the cruise, and the mood lifts.

The passengers forgive and forget the drama of spending the first night in port with a school-dinner-type meal, and all the pools on board are gloriously warm, making swimming in them an absolute dream. Plus, the crew brew up some patriotic festivities. Union Jack flags flutter in the breeze, accompanied by the lively chatter of passengers enjoying Pimm's, setting the stage for a vibrant deck party.

Laughter and cheers permeate the air. A dance competition begins with the infectious beats of "Celebrate Good Times" and "YMCA" energising the crowd. Don and I showcase our disco moves, incorporating the wheelchair seamlessly into our routine. It's pretty bonkers, but great fun. We win first prize—a free cocktail each.

Another perk is that there's a Costa Coffee on board. We have to pay extra if we want to indulge in this treat, and for some years now we've been into speciality and artisan coffees, so we invest in one of the Costa Coffee prepaid cards.

A few years previously, we'd visited a working men's club in Birmingham for a cheap and cheerful brunch with my family, and Don ordered a *Latte* at the bar. The bloke serving us looked at Don quizzically, as if he were from another planet, completely baffled by his request, and my nephew, Dan, split his sides laughing.

'A lar-tay?!' Dan mimicked Don's pronunciation of "*Latte*". 'You won't get a lar-tay in 'ere, Don!'

Just then, my sister walked into the working men's club as

we were ordering our drinks.

'Hey Mom,' continued Dan, still doubled up with laughter, 'Don's just ordered a lar-tay!'

My sister giggled at the incongruity. Trust Don to ask for a speciality coffee in a working men's club. He wasn't impressed that he had to make do with a cheap brand of instant coffee to accompany his brunch instead.

The *Oriana* ship is an old lady now.

With my penchant for enjoying a few ship facts, I discovered she was the first cruise ship commissioned for P&O cruises and entered into service in April 1995. She'd been refurbished in 2011, and there are just over 900 cabins, nearly 2000 passengers, and 800 crew.

She's powered by four diesel engines. Despite her being 20 years old (the same age as Tim who doesn't come with us on this trip), she's still rather elegant, particularly in the speciality dining restaurant where we pay a supplement one evening to sample some exclusive culinary delights. The food is, without a doubt, a notch up there.

As usual, I get lost on the ship. My sense of direction has never been good and I always confuse the front and the back of the vessel, but I discover that on the *Oriana* the casino is like a compass and I have to pass through this part of the ship many times to get to our cabin.

It's an eye-opener.

I've never set foot in a casino before and it's an alien environment to me (though oddly enough, when I was in my teens, I was keen to train as a croupier. I'd have been hopeless at the job!). The casino is continually busy, and it must rake in tens of thousands of pounds for P&O as the punters play morning, noon and night. I conclude they must be either extremely wealthy, or getting into a lot of debt.

Our cruise itinerary takes us to two places we'd visited

before—Gibraltar (where I'm pleased to find that the watch lady in the pop-up stall is still there, and I buy a couple more) and Lisbon. But we also visit some fresh places: Cadiz, Malaga and La Coruna.

At Lisbon, we give the whining *Ponte 25 de Abril* a miss and Don braves the cobblestones in search of a pale blue scarf. He's seen a man on the ship wearing one and he thinks it looks very smart. This time I'm in sensible shoes suitable for the cobbles.

Don is like a dog with a bone in search of a pale blue scarf and he's determined to buy one in Lisbon to remind him of the place. We come across several, but at around 30 euros they're too expensive for him.

Then, as we're about to give up, we discover a tiny cheap stall just off the square which has one for only 6 euros. It's perfect for him. He also buys his first selfie stick. *Boys and their toys.*

There's some kind of love-fest going on in the city square. Countless tiny metal hearts, adorned with tender declarations of love by those who have written on them, have been securely fastened onto a colossal framework of towering letters that spell out L O V E. I pick up a heart and a marker, and I can't resist adding to the number.

After a while, the cobblestones play havoc with Don's insides, so we catch a tram and explore further afield. This time we enjoyed our visit to Lisbon much more than our cashless visit in 2008 and finally got to savour a Bica coffee.

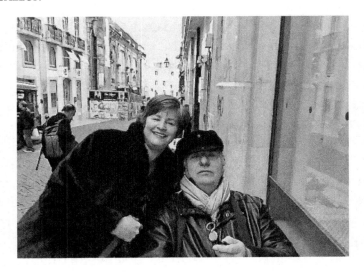

Lisbon - Don modelling his 6 euro pale blue
scarf using the selfie stick

The charming ports of Cadiz, Malaga, and La Coruna delight us as we navigate these places at our own pace, opting out of paid excursions. The mere pleasure of basking in the cool shade of the main square, savouring a crisp glass of wine and relishing the tangy aroma of olives, is satisfaction enough for us.

There was a talent show aboard this cruise and having honed my skills as a hotel pianist for a couple of years, I signed up to play a captivating piano cover of *Moon River* arranged by the talented Philip Keveren. A man in the audience so loved the arrangement, he took down the details so he could play it himself back home. Mind you, the musical offerings of all the participants paled with the last act: a fabulous female vocalist who flawlessly belted out an unforgettable performance of *Simply The Best*. She could have been Tina Turner herself, so phenomenal was her rendition.

All in all, it is a pleasant cruise and excellent value for money once again at less than £100 per person per day, but now for the journey home.

I'm dreading it.

The worst part is getting our luggage from the port to Southampton Central Station. We still skimp and scrape and decide not to take an accessible taxi, so we have a long 45-minute walk ahead. Don is off in his electric wheelchair, brolly in one hand, steering his chair with the other, bags piled high on his knees.

'Follow me,' he commands, waving his brolly.

It's hard keeping up with him at the best of times, but he's way ahead of me as I rumble our two cases on wheels after him.

And then I lose him.

At the end of an endless road, he's disappeared.

Where the hell is he?

I don't know whether to turn right or left. This often happens if we're out around the town shopping. One minute he's behind me, then I turn around and he's gone. But this was a straight path.

I ring his mobile.

No answer.

I try several times, leaving a message.

No answer.

This isn't happening to me—we travel hundreds of miles and lose each other in Southampton.

Then I see him coming towards me with his folded umbrella up in the air waving at me, all perky.

'Where have you been?' he asks.

'I can't walk that fast! You disappeared,' I whine.

'Our train leaves soon, follow me!' he does an about-turn and off he goes again as I trot after him, pushing our cases as fast as I can. We just about make it in time.

'That's it. I never want to go on a cruise again!' I sulk as I slump into my train seat, exhausted from all the exertion. 'And I can't cope with all this luggage!'

Tanty over, Don gets out his laptop and I de-stress by

listening to some Bach on my iPod.

No, never again. That's it. I'm not doing any more cruises.

Moon River - arranged by Philip Keveren

83. SIXTIETH BIRTHDAY TREAT

'Are you married?' asks Suzi, my *Adore Your Pelvic Floor* teacher.

'Yes,' I nod.

'To a man?'

It's June 2018 and I'm in the quirky town of Totnes (the sort of place where, as a woman, you're not surprised to be asked if you're married to a man) at a pelvic floor class exploring the whys and wherefores of keeping well-toned in that area of one's anatomy. But it's because of this class that my wanderlust returns somewhat.

There are only three of us in the "Adore Your (pelvic) Floor" class. There's me plus one other pupil, Christine, along with our tutor Suzi, who gives us lots of advice about embracing the challenges of the menopause. She teaches us how to do Kegels[1] properly. You see, you can't just squeeze your arse any old how. There's a special way to do pelvic floor exercises and they have to be taught and then practised. Not only that, there are different kinds of pelvic floor squeezes, including The Knack[2] for when you sneeze, cough, or lift something heavy. It's quite complicated.

On the flip side, Suzi also teaches us how to relax the pelvic floor area and we find that much harder than learning the squeezes.

'It's important to restore a balanced tone to the pelvic floor area,' Suzi encourages us. 'Pelvic floor care isn't all about the squeezes.'

I learned more about the anatomy of my body in these

classes than I ever did at school.

On the way to our cars after the class, Christine tells me about her recent cruise to the Fjords and how beautiful and majestic they are. My 60th birthday is on the horizon in June 2019. It gives me an idea: a cruise to the Fjords would be a lovely birthday treat. *I wonder if it's still only £100 per person per day for an inside cabin?*

Despite some of my ill-at-ease feelings with cruises, I surrender to the fact that they are still the best way for Don and me to see some of the world and that they are also excellent value for money. They're still much cheaper than full-board for seven nights in a hotel in the UK. Not only that, cruise ships cater exceptionally well for wheelchair users.

I also fancy sailing north rather than travelling to a hot and sunny country. Don loves the sun however, and he's a tad disappointed with my suggestion (he's also not keen on crossing the North Sea with his sea sickness issues), but in 2017 I was diagnosed with three stage zero ("in situ") malignant melanomas which had to be surgically removed. My medical team advised me to stay out of the sun to reduce the chance of any more malignant moles developing. A cooler climate would be perfect.

The next day I find a cruise to the Fjords from the 1st to the 8th of June 2019, which is splendid as my birthday is on the 4th of June. I book it there and then with P&O Cruises. We always have to book at least a year in advance because people snatch up the accessible cabins almost as soon as the cruise goes live.

We'll be aboard the Azura cruise liner—seven nights for £649 per person in an accessible cabin, with an "obstructed" porthole. *Good-oh.*

[1] *Pelvic Floor Exercises*

[2] *The Knack is a skill to contract the pelvic floor muscles before an increase in abdominal pressure, such as when coughing, sneezing or lifting.*

84. NORWEGIAN FJORDS 2019

While booking the cruise over the phone, I make an interesting discovery: Cunard and P&O are part of the same parent company—Carnival. We would have liked to have sailed on the beautiful *Queen Mary 2* again, but it was more expensive than P&O.

On learning that P&O and Cunard are sister companies, I whine and moan to the booking assistant and I explain to her that our Cunard cruise had been extremely disappointing with the awful annexe cabin. I tell her we do not want a repeat experience of that.

Then she surprises me.

As a gesture of goodwill, they give us an extra $100 each for onboard spending as compensation (even though it happened nearly ten years ago) because they are part of the same parent company, Carnival Cruises.

It makes my day.

On the downside, we have to travel by train because our price does not include parking. Again. *Never say never!*

This time I refuse point blank to cart all our luggage from Southampton Central Station to the port, so we fork out for an accessible taxi.

We have to wait 45 minutes for a cab that Don can get his electric wheelchair into. *We could have blummin' well walked it in that time.* But it was worth the wait.

Our friends from Birmingham, Mike and Hoa, join us on the cruise (the name "Hoa" means "flower"). Mike met Hoa when she came to Britain as one of the Vietnamese Boat People. She is Hoa by name and Hoa by nature as she loves flowers and gardening, and we're both enamoured with the spectacular and most beautiful stems that adorn all the dining tables. I download an App on my phone which will recognise a bloom and discover it is an *Ornithogalum umbellatum* (Star of Bethlehem).

Our itinerary embraces strange-sounding names and faraway places: Stavanger, Flåm, Alesund. My father would have loved those names. Unusual-sounding words fascinated him.

On the 4th of June, I get a birthday card from the captain and his crew. How kind. The ship takes notes of the passengers' date of birth. *Nice touch!*

The Captain's "Notes from the Bridge" for the 4th of June 2019 on the *Azura* demonstrate that navigating a cruise liner through a fjord is not as straightforward as it might seem...

Tuesday 4 June 2019 - Flåm

The Captain, Trevor Lane, arrived on the Bridge at 12.45 am ready to assist the Bridge Officers with the fjord transit. The Pilot also arrived shortly afterwards and 'the conn' of the vessel was handed to him for the entrance to the fjord. The run into Flåm is widely regarded as one of the longest most breathtaking transits that can be experienced on a ship of Azura's size. This marked the beginning of a 100-nautical mile journey until Azura reached her berth at the end of the fjord.

Azura was on her final approach to the village of Flåm at 6.30 am and the Deputy Captain arrived on the Bridge for the arrival. The vessel came starboard side alongside the cruise pier in Flåm with the Deputy Captain carrying out the manoeuvre. It took the mooring teams longer than usual to tie up the vessel due to the short nature of the quay. However, the vessel was all fast by 7.45 am and guests were able to go ashore by 8.00 am.

At 5.08 pm, all guests and crew were back on board and the ship was ready to put to sea. All lines were gone by 5.43 pm and this allowed the Deputy Captain to thrust the vessel clear of the berth and set the engines astern. Once the vessel reached the swinging circle, he used Azura's bow thrusters to swing the ship around to starboard, lining the vessel up on a reciprocal track as the one used for the arrival. With the towering fjord cliffs on either side, Azura set off on her 100-mile journey out of Sognafjord (South Fjord). At 11.38 pm, Azura exited the fjord making her way into the North Sea and proceeding further North towards Alesund.

Weather: Overcast with occasional breaks in cloud
Temperature: 16° C
Wind: Light airs

After our evening meal, I'm in a celebratory mood.

I fancy a bop at the late-night disco to conclude my birthday. We usually enjoy a dance together, Don and I, and we're pretty darn good at wheelchair dancing. But tonight Don feels conked out, so I go on my own and join in with the ravers —mature people my age having a fantastic time. We're all approaching the last lap of life, conscious that time is running out, so we give it some welly.

Then, a female singer and live band comes on and strikes up a great boppy-type riff. I don't recognise the melody at all, but it has an excellent beat for dancing. Then, out of the blue, everyone is singing at the top of their voices about a woman called Eileen.

'Come on Eileen!' they chorus. 'Come on Eileen!'

Eileen?

Who is Eileen? What is she?

How do they all know this song? Have I missed something?

They sing it with gusto, like they're at a football match, and wave their arms about like they're at Glastonbury. They're having a ball. I'm standing there dumb in the middle of the crowd as I don't know the words or the tune, so I call it a night and head off to bed.

85. AN EXCURSION AT LAST!

On the 6th of June, we visit Bergen and I go on my first-ever cruise ship excursion with Mike and Hoa, and it is worth paying the extra money to experience it.

It's a trip to Troldhaugen—the home of the famous composer Edward Greig, who built the house and lived there from 1885 until he died in 1907.

I'm fascinated to visit the place where his musical inspiration flourished. As I wander through his house and behold all his accoutrements and pictures, I get a genuine sense of his creativity, but I'm shocked to discover he'd married his first cousin (Nina). I guess it was a different time and different place back then.

The excursion includes an amazing concert in the spectacular concert hall, which has a breathtaking view of the garden behind the piano.

The pianist, Knut Christian Jansson, is excellent, and he plays "Wedding Day at Troldhaugen" to perfection on the beautiful Steinway grand piano. This challenging and complex composition by Grieg holds special memories for me because Don and I played this jaunty descriptive piece as a duet at our wedding reception to entertain our guests in 1994.

The concert concludes with a piano arrangement of the song "Modersorg" (A Mother's Grief). It is even more poignant having learnt that Grieg and his wife Nina lost their only child to meningitis in 1868.

Don cannot come with us because the excursion is not

suitable for wheelchair users. Instead, he takes a ride on Fløibanen, Bergen's Funicular Railway, up to the top of Mount Fløyen and he has a grand time on his own (well, apart from waiting two hours to get on the train, that is).

Our excursion to Troldhaugen is a great success, despite losing Mike after the concert. He's a keen photographer and disappears into the undergrowth of the garden with his trusty camera. Then, like David Attenborough, he re-emerges just as we are about to head back for the ship. *Good timing.*

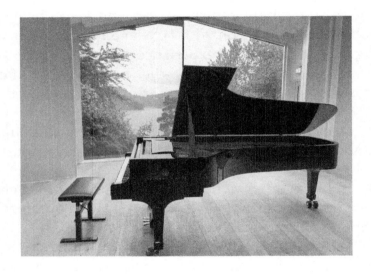

Concert hall at Troldhaugen

It's lovely having Mike (who insists on calling Don "Donald") and Hoa join us on the cruise. Don knew them both for many years before we married. Mike is in sympathy with me over certain aspects of cruising, which he also finds distasteful, and I sense it is likely to be their first and last cruise.

Our voyage was smooth sailing in every way, both on the sea and aboard - apart that is from the onboard pools being rather chilly and unheated, making my daily swim uncomfortable. Oh, and the long queues at meal times, plus the fact that Don seems to know several passengers on the cruise. I find this rather irritating and the phrase "what a small world" is a frequent mantra of ours on this trip. He bumps into many couples he knows from his various pursuits and interests in the UK. *Far out!* Don often meets friends almost everywhere we go in the UK. But on a cruise ship in the Fjords? It was uncanny.

Toward the end of the cruise, we pay for a special tour of the kitchens, culminating in an outstanding lunch. It's fascinating to learn how the chefs cater for thousands of people on a cruise liner. I've never seen such enormous kitchen bowls and mixers in all my days.

Stunning displays of mouth-watering food and intricate carvings of melons and various fruits adorn the tour. The tantalising aroma of freshly baked bread envelops us, showcasing the skill of the bakers who prepare it fresh on board every day. *No wonder it tastes so good.*

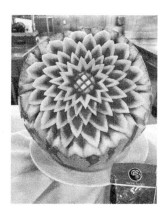

A carved melon

We decide to experience the Sunday morning service. I'm

intrigued and fascinated by this event and how the Captain and his officers lead these conventional services, which are always very dignified. Underpinning this ritual are centuries of spiritual naval tradition.

On this occasion, however, I'm beguiled by the pianist accompanying the congregation as they joyfully sing the traditional Anglican hymns. I can see the concentration etched on his face as he navigates through unfamiliar chords and melodies. He's not acquainted with any of the hymns, it seems, as he meticulously sight-reads the sheet music, leaning in so close that his nose almost touches the paper, determined not to miss a note. He looks quite comical.

I sympathise with him though. Hymns are not as easy to play as you would imagine, and as a wedding organist, I knew only too well how tricky they can be. I'd struggle myself to sight-read many of the hymns he was playing.

A few hours later, I see him happily playing a keyboard for the ballroom dances with a small band. He needs no music at all and is completely at home free-wheeling the keys. I guess the life of a cruise pianist can have its twists and turns.

Our cruise to the Fjords has been a delightful experience and a perfect way to celebrate my six decades on planet Earth. Thank you P&O Cruises for a lovely time.

Less than a year later, the world of cruising came to a halt during the Covid pandemic.

Our only link to cruising was to see several liners moored in Torbay for many months during this time. We felt for the crew who were keeping them ticking over.

The liners became our silent friends during the lockdowns —a companion of memories past and beacons of hope for the future, that they would, one day, sail again with guests aboard.

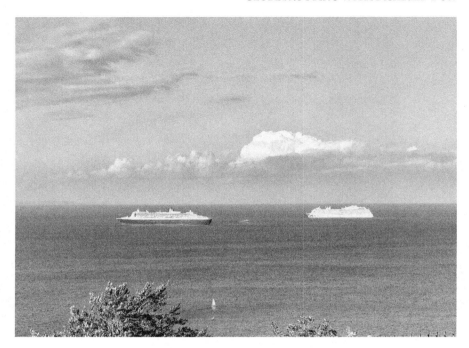

Liners in Torbay during the Covid pandemic.
They were there for many months.

PART EIGHT - DOES BRITAIN COUNT?

English Escapades

86. STAYCATION ANECDOTES

In between our travels abroad, there have been several trips and holidays in Britain (with and without Tim depending on his age), and the following anecdotes sum up the flavour and nature of our experiences. Some are related to Don's disability and the difficulties that presents to us (including my role as his carer), some are related to his personality traits, and some are just stuff that can happen to anyone. But all of them are true and reflect the unpredictability of travel, and life in general, at times.

CORNWALL 1999

'Tim's very wheezy Don, his asthma's playing up,' I observe, concerned that the inhaler we use isn't working.

It's late on a Saturday night, and we find ourselves nestled in a beautifully quaint and picturesque farmhouse bed and breakfast in deepest, darkest Cornwall, with four-year-old Tim. The asthma doesn't settle down and gets worse. I know we need a hospital where he can go on a more powerful ventilator.

At 3 a.m. we decide to go to the hospital. After getting dressed, we make tracks, though not before the door knob drops off and clatters noisily onto the floorboards, setting off the farm dogs barking furiously. We make a speedy exit and drive off towards Penzance, the nearest town where there's an Accident & Emergency.

The deserted country lanes are pitch black and we make

good time.

It's almost 4 a.m. when we hit Penzance and I'm completely taken aback at the sight that greets us.

87. BRIGHT YOUNG THINGS

The place is heaving with life.

Hoards of young people are out on the town, drinking, dancing, laughing.

It's buzzing.

We have a job driving through the crowds crisscrossing the main street, slowing down to a snail's pace.

'Crikey, to think all this goes on while we're tucked up in bed snoring our heads off every Saturday at 4 o'clock in the morning,' I observe.

We finally make it through and pull up at the hospital.

'Well, I could have understood the hold-up if we'd been slap bang in the middle of Birmingham city centre! But Penzance?' I quiz.

The hospital sorts out Tim and we're back in bed by 7 a.m. to catch an hour of kip. We then enjoy a fabulous Cornish breakfast of bacon, sausage, egg, hogs pudding[1], and gorgeous toasted homemade bread - all local ingredients served by our lovely hostess at her kitchen table.

I wasn't able to fix the doorknob, so I came clean about it and explained what had happened during the night.

'Yes, I heard you drive off and the dogs barking. Don't worry about it. I'm just pleased your son is OK now,' is her gracious response.

Gosh, I bet she thought we'd done a bunk without paying. I wouldn't blame her.

I often think of Penzance teeming with Bright Young Things,

heaving with life on Saturday nights. Where *did* they all go?

[1] *A traditional Cornish sausage made to a special recipe.*

88. THOSE MAGNIFICENT MEN IN THEIR FLYING MACHINES

It's a beautiful summer day on the 24th of August 2000 and the atmosphere is buzzing with excitement at the Dartmouth Regatta in Devon.

The Red Arrows will showcase not only their magnificent jets but also their skill and precision with formation flying, culminating in a death-defying stunt where they fly low over the River Dart. One jet flies to the right, passing another jet flying to the left, in the opposite direction.

They just miss each other.

It's a perfect occasion to have a family day out, especially as Dartmouth is only a few miles from our home. I pack a picnic barbecue, and we arrive early to get a good view. Five-year-old Tim is excited to see the Red Arrows at such close range.

The clear blue sky stretches overhead and soon the pavement is six deep. A sense of anticipation surrounds us as the spectators eagerly await the thrilling display of skill and precision by the amazing pilots, looping the loop and defying the ground.

It's 5.30 p.m. and there's another half hour to go before the Red Arrows appear at 6 p.m. The late August weather is hot —just perfect for the planes. We've carted our barbecue picnic with us, and I assume we'll choose a pleasant spot somewhere after the show to cook the food, but Don has other ideas.

Don is hungry.

He sets up the portable barbecue.

'You can't cook it here!' I pooh-pooh, surrounded by crowds of people.

'It's fine, darling, nobody will mind. You worry too much.'

And so it was that Don cooked a barbecue right in the middle of a crowd watching the Red Arrows at Dartmouth Regatta. The deafening roar of their magnificent engines reverberated through the air, while their red, white and blue smoke trails mingled with the smoke rising from our chicken and burgers.

Don was right—nobody batted an eyelid. But I really didn't enjoy the experience!

89. BIRMINGHAM

It's late summer, 2008, and we're on one of our frequent travels to Birmingham to visit family.

Both Don and I were born in Birmingham and still have relatives living there. We're staying in a Travelodge at the Maypole, about seven miles south of the city centre. We got a special value deal at only £9 a night midweek rate for a family room, which includes a bed pulled out from under the sofa for thirteen-year-old Tim.

Walking towards Primrose (my nickname for our Mercedes Sprinter van) in the car park, we see myriads of tiny pieces of glass scattered all around her, shining like diamonds in the morning sun. It's a telltale sign that there's been a break-in.

The window on the driver's side has been smashed and there's glass everywhere, both inside and outside our vehicle.

It's a mess.

Someone has stolen our sat nav. How stupid of us to leave it in full view.

I'd bought the sat nav, a TomTom, after we'd got hopelessly lost trying to find Leicester and almost ended up in Lincoln. It was a birthday present for Don and he was NOT impressed with it at first because he loves maps. But he soon warmed to it (even though it took us down a dirt track to a dead end once, as they do), and we rely heavily on it.

'Why did you leave the sat nav on display in the window?' I quiz Don, though truth be told we're both responsible.

'I forgot. It never crossed my mind anyone would want to steal a TomTom. I guess they stole it to sell for cash.'

Then I saw Don's Nokia mobile phone on the dashboard next

to where the TomTom had been.

'Well, would you believe it? You left your mobile right there as well, but they haven't touched that. They missed a trick there!'

We return to the Travelodge and report the crime to them, but they can't do a thing about it. 'Parking is at your own risk,' they say. *Fair enough.*

I clean up as much of the shattered glass as I can and Don goes into the Wilko store next to the Travelodge to get some sticky tape and black bags so I can patch up the broken window. He comes back feeling very pleased with himself as he's explained to the cashier what's happened and he learns Wilko has security cameras positioned over the car park.

'The staff in Wilko are fantastic,' he enthuses. 'They're looking through the film right now. I'm going back to see what they've found.'

The security staff at Wilko found the relevant film - Don watches the thieves smash our window and steal the sat nav. Great! Now we have video evidence. Don contacts the police and lets them know.

But the police aren't interested whatsoever and do sod all about this petty crime. *Oh well.* "If that's all that happens to you in life, you'll get by," I can hear my mother's voice say. True enough.

I loved that TomTom. I particularly liked the voice of "Tim" who spoke with a plumb in his mouth - he was wonderfully calming. We buy a Garmin to replace it, but the male voice is nowhere near as sexy as the voice of Tim the TomTom-man.

While we're in Birmingham, we pay a visit to our friends Mike and Hoa who live in Handsworth, and afterwards, we go into the city centre to do some shopping. We head to the ShopMobility booth so that Don can hire a scooter, only to find he's been banned from using them because he'd crashed one of the ShopMobility scooters in Torquay into a shop front several months previously. He's been blacklisted. So that was the end of that.

To cap it all on our way back home, I have a strop. It happened like this: we're careering down the M5 and without warning, Don turns off towards Weston-Super-Mare.

'Where are you going?' I enquire.

'I thought it'd be nice to visit Weston on our way home.' Don has a soft spot for Weston as he'd lived there briefly.

'But I don't want to go to Weston.'

'Well, I do. It's a lovely place.'

'I know it is, but I've got all the unpacking to do when I get home and time's getting on. How long will it take to get there?'

'It's only twenty minutes or so.'

'And twenty minutes back, and then at least half an hour there. It's extending our journey home by nearly an hour and a half!' I whine.

Don does an about-turn at a roundabout and heads back home, sacrificing the pleasure trip to Weston.

Under different circumstances, it would have been nice to have had a diversion there, but sometimes my anxiety kicks in and I'm always thinking about the next task at hand. I'm eager to unpack, put everything in its place and get the dirty clothes in the washing machine. If I'd been more laid back, the diversion wouldn't have affected me, especially as at the time I wasn't working and had the next day free. So now, when I feel the anxiety creeping up, I always ask Don, 'Can we please go straight home without any detours?'

But in recent years, having learnt to be more chilled, I'm occasionally up for a wee diversion on the way home if the day is still young...

90. THE NATIONAL TRUST

We are members of the National Trust and we like to get our money's worth from our membership. If we pass fairly close to a National Trust property on our way home from holiday, I'm often up for a deviation in our journey - especially as I've learnt to chill out a bit more.

Wonderful grounds and gorgeous gardens frequently adorn these properties, as well as an interesting shop and cafés selling delicious homemade cakes, along with the opportunity to nose around someone's stately (or sometimes not-so-stately) home. What's not to like?

So once, on our way back from Wales, we stop off at a property to savour the delightful atmosphere that's very often instilled in these quintessential British places. We head straight for the café, as we're both in need of refreshments and once we're fortified with homemade carrot cake and a flat white coffee, we set off to explore the grand house.

Don discovers the upstairs is not accessible, so I go mooching up there on my own and take photographs to show him later, and then we go around the ground floor inspecting the fascinating kitchens with all the old pots and pans and other Victorian kitchenware.

I always love the old kitchens the best, I'm not sure why. I try to visualise it in its heyday with cooks and servants all busily doing their tasks as I attempt to conjure up the smells, the sounds, the sights, and the food - not all of them perhaps palatable to my sanitised experience of food in the 20th and

21st centuries.

We move on to other rooms. There's a piano in one room and guests are permitted to play it. There's a book of Chopin Waltzes, so I play the one in A-flat which is my "go-to" Chopin Waltz. What a treat! Sometimes guests are allowed to play instruments at National Trust properties, sometimes not. I'm disappointed to discover that guests cannot play the harpsichord in the drawing room, but then that's perfectly understandable as they're more delicate instruments.

Next is the enormous dining room. The long table is beautifully laid out with much ornate crockery, cutlery and glassware. I visualise all the lords and ladies dining in their finery. What gossip and conversations could these walls tell?

Then we're through to the large lounge, where the walls are covered in paintings of dead people. Who are they? What were their loves and their hates? So much history.

I look at my watch. Try as I might to be more laid back, I'm still conscious of time. It's getting on and I have to unpack quite a lot of things.

'I think we should head for home soon, darling. Shall we glance at the gardens quickly?' I say to Don. He twirls around in his six-wheeled electric wheelchair to exit the room, but one wheel catches an ancient rug and drags it along, whereupon it gets all tangled up as he spins back and forth, trying to extricate himself.

I am horrified.

'Don, don't move! You're making it worse!' I hiss, trying not to draw attention to the predicament.

Thankfully, there isn't a Room Guide around to witness this spectacle. Two more visitors, a man and a woman, enter the room, whereupon the man helps Don disentangle his wheels from the carpet, which is now all scrunched up. Hopefully, it will recover from its ordeal.

We make a speedy escape to the gardens with profuse thanks to our rescuer.

91. SALCOMBE

'C'mon, we're not made of sugar!' Don remarks, getting his own back at me for using this phrase I often use at him when I remind him that a bit of rain won't hurt him. But this time he means it as he and Tim unload the blow-up boat from Primrose, our van.

This boat is a serious piece of kit, complete with a Yamaha engine. It's no kiddy toy. It cost £500 out of our re-mortgage money, and Don is determined to give the boat a whirl. We've spent the day in Salcombe, and we're at the North Sands beach. The tide is in, perfect!

Tim is a strapping young teenager and can handle the job, no problem. The cool, damp August weather has been dodgy all day, making our picnic lunch rather grim. Plus, it was too windy for my liking, but glimpses of the sun peeking through the brisk clouds had brought out several families to enjoy a breezy Sunday afternoon on the beach.

We park up right opposite the beach just as everyone packs up and goes home. A large black cloud is looming, threatening a downpour.

This does not deter Don, and he orders Tim, who's a willing accomplice in this boating fest, as he unloads it and sets it all up ready to launch.

'I don't think this is a good idea at all,' I quip. 'It's going to tip down with rain soon. I think we should go home like everyone else. I want a cup of tea.'

'But me and Tim want to do it. Tim, get the engine,' orders Don.

A big raindrop falls just as Tim drags the boat onto the beach.

Then another and another.

'I told you it's going to rain. And I'm cold. I want to go home,' I whine.

I sit in the relative warmth of the car, having a tanty, refusing to help. *Let them get on with it.*

More raindrops fall, quicker this time, just as they attempt to launch. It's a struggle for Don, who uses his arm crutches supported by Tim, but he's determined to get a boat ride in.

Soon there's a deluge and they have to make a hasty retreat. They both get drenched as they dismantle the boat engine, take out all the air, pack it away in a rather higgledy-piggledy fashion, and stuff it into the back of the van.

We drive home.

If only they'd listened to me.

Fast forward to 2021. It's 6 a.m. and I open the curtains of the rear side window of Primrose, our van. We've slept overnight at North Sands seafront, and from the comfort of the double bed which Don had built into the back of our vehicle (literally a soft mattress on a board over the boot, nothing fancy), we watch a woman and her dog paddle-board over to Salcombe Harbour.

Idyllic.

What a lovely thing to do.

It gives me a perspective of myself that I've missed something in life.

It's a glorious morning and already warm at 7 a.m. Lockdown is becoming a distant memory as life gets back to normal.

Things are good.

I help Don get dressed, and he decides he'd like a shave in the van. Even though there's a decent disabled toilet across the road, he's determined to experience his shaving ablutions from the comfort of his vehicle and he's brought all his shaving accoutrements with him. How lovely to have a morning shave by the sea. I give him a bowl of water. But it's a disaster and there's shaving foam everywhere. It's on the dashboard, the steering wheel, on the window and there are large drips of it all down his nice clean blue T-shirt. He does look a mess.

If you've ever tried to get shaving foam off a cotton T-shirt, you will know it's an impossible task. I make a mental note to buy him an electric shaver for his birthday.

'I think you should give shaving in the van a miss in future!' I advise. 'I'll get the kettle on.'

We get out of the van to enjoy the sunshine and I set up our little calor gas stove on a low wall flanking the field opposite the beach. We need our morning cuppa.

I light the stove, but I'm completely unprepared for what happens next.

92. IT AIN'T HALF HOT MUM

There's a big WHOOSH!

Flames engulf the stove, flaring up lustily ten or twelve inches.

I narrowly avoid getting my hair and eyebrows singed and stand back aghast, staring at it in disbelief, as do Don and a group of paddle-boarding youths nearby who are entranced by this fire drama, sniggering. *How embarrassing.*

A man appears from nowhere.

'Have you got a towel?' he asks calmly. I grab one out of the van and he puts out the fire by throwing it over the flames.

He has a dog and was walking across the field on the other side of the wall just as he witnessed the fire ignite and came to help us while we gawped helplessly at the blaze. How kind.

Don immediately starts chatting with this helpful stranger, extracting his entire life story (which has not been a happy one) in less than ten minutes flat. The man also owns a small camper van, which co-incidentally is parked right behind our vehicle. Don notices the solar panels on it and spends half an hour quizzing the man about this solar device. He wonders whether they might be powerful enough to charge up his electric wheelchair. The man says no. *Dream on Don.* They're great for living life off-grid, though, he said.

We then head to the town centre for a cooked breakfast. And a cup of tea.

93. HOLIDAY AT HOME

One year we tried a "holiday at home".

It didn't work.

I was run ragged doing washing, ironing, answering emails, phone calls and doing all the normal chores while trying to pack picnics nearly every day.

It was exhausting. *Never again.*

It's at the beginning of one of these "holiday at home" days that Don has a hissy fit over his mobile phone, which goes missing.

'Where's my mobile? I can't remember when I had it last,' Don calls to me from the bedroom.

It's early in the morning and he's drinking a cuppa in bed while I get some breakfast and organise the picnic food.

'I don't know where it is.' *Gordon Bennett, there's always summat.* Constant interruptions are a given when one is a carer.

'Can you ring it please?' he implores.

'OK, but it's probably on silent as usual.'

We often have conversations like this while we're in separate rooms. It's just how it is with us.

I ring his mobile from mine.

Nothing.

I look everywhere for it. First in the van, but it's not there. Then I look in all of Don's bags (no mean feat as he has several and I never know what's lurking at the bottom of them), then I scour through all his pockets (no mean feat again as bits of food and sticky sweets are usually stuck in them). Finally, I look in his bathroom, but it's nowhere to be seen.

'I'm really worried about my mobile. I think I lost it up the field when I was flying my kite. I've got to go up there and look for it. Can you get me up, please?'

'OK, OK, I'm coming.'

I drop what I'm doing, and get a bowl of warm water, a flannel, a towel and some aqueous cream with a few drops of tea tree oil on it (which is very good for fending off infections). For some years I've been helping Don with his morning ablutions in this way because for him to take a shower every day isn't as simple as one would think, particularly if he has any broken skin on his feet where an infection can get in through any soiled shower water. Even the tiniest break in the skin can get infected if bacteria enter it and cause very painful cellulitis. Don has been in hospital with infections too many times and knows how debilitating they are.

We also find that doing a daily bed bath keeps urine infections at bay. I'm used to it and pleased to do it because it only takes a few minutes and we've had excellent results with this regime. It works well for us. It has improved Don's health no end, eliminating the need for regular use of antibiotics.

So with everything prepared to do a bed bath, I lift the appropriate body part and I gasp.

94. GOOD VIBRATIONS

There, underneath his private bits, is his mobile phone (I kid you not!)

'Blummin' heck, here's your mobile under your willy! Didn't you feel it vibrate when I rang it?'

'No?' is the questioning response from Don as if he should have.

'I don't believe it! How on earth did it get *there?!*'

'I don't know, but what a relief. I'm so pleased we've found it.'

I laugh, but Don doesn't see the funny side as he's too overwhelmed by relief that it's been found, particularly as it's in a case with his credit and debit cards. I wipe the phone well.

While he's still lying on the bed, I pull on his socks, then underpants (always socks before underpants to avoid introducing infection to the groin area from the feet - a tip we learnt off the internet), then a pair of long johns, followed by his trousers and finally his shoes. Then he sits up and grabs the chest of drawers next to the bed to haul himself up so that I can pull everything up. I notice his phone charging wire is stuck to his left buttock. *Good grief, what has he been doing with that phone!* Proving that if it can happen, it will.

'Thank you,' he says as I pull up his underpants.

'Thank you,' he says as I pull up his long johns.

'Thank you,' he says as I pull up his trousers.

It's extremely helpful as a carer when the person you care for is thankful, and Don excels in this gift. He's always exceedingly grateful for any help I give him, and this makes for a good relationship between the carer and the cared-for.

Then Don goes off to do bowel irrigation and a wee—but he does a wee using intermittent self-catheterisation.

Self-catheterisation has transformed the lives of many disabled people. However, at first, Don had to exercise some self-advocacy as his urologist was very much against it due to the risks it could carry. But Don persevered, and he is so much better as a result of being able to empty his bladder thoroughly using this technique. Besides that, self-catheterisation has improved over the years, reducing the risks involved.

There are now also self-catheterisation units with bags attached which are portable and can be used anywhere and everywhere as well as during the night.

Don sometimes uses the ones with a bag on the end and I'm often surprised at how much urine it holds - it's almost full at 1400ml. I'd be in absolute agony if my bladder had to hold that much. Don's neuropathic bladder must swell to the size of a small balloon. But a doctor once told him it's good that his bladder is so elastic. The problems begin, the doctor explained, when bladders go hard and won't expand, so I guess 1400ml is encouraging.

I get back to finishing my jobs, dovetailing several chores to maximise time. It's a beautiful day, and we later enjoy a picnic in one of our local favourite beauty spots—Battery Gardens in Brixham.

On the subject of Don and his kites, quite simply, he loves the things and often carries one around in his bag. He'll attempt to fly it anywhere at any time and will rope in anyone who will help him get it off the ground.

I now flatly refuse to be his kite-thrower-upper since a somewhat embarrassing incident at Llandudno seafront (I should point out Don was 77 when this took place).

It happened like this: Don loves to mooch around the cheap

and cheerful shops lining one of Llandudno's main streets and he buys a kite for £1. We head for the seafront and he's eager to try it out straight away.

'You can't fly your kite here!' I beseech.

'It'll be fine, darling, you worry too much. Help me unravel the string and then throw it up in the air. There's a lovely sea breeze.'

After several attempts, we get it off the ground and Don does a quick spurt in his electric wheelchair along the promenade so that the velocity kicks in to keep it flying. It's a jazzy little kite with a rainbow-coloured tail, but within seconds it goes into a nosedive, spiralling erratically.

I'm mortified as I watch it descend, powerless to stop this fearsome toy from wreaking its havoc. I look on helplessly as the kite plummets and hits a man on the head, then the string floats down and gets tangled around a dog, and finally strings across a family having a picnic on the beach. Oddly enough, everyone seems to think it's rather funny, including the man whose head took a knock. Don strikes up a conversation with him, extracting his life story in ten minutes flat. As he does.

That's when I made the mental note to disown Don the next time he gets his kite out in public.

But dramas occurred even if we went nowhere—especially if Harold, Don's father, was around.

Harold could be dreadfully accident-prone and often got into a pickle, whether it was driving his mobility scooter down a ditch in Churston as the afternoon sun made him sleepy under the plastic canopy (along with the effects of a very large lunch and two halves of mild at his local pub), or the frequent occasions when he fell over in his bungalow, whereupon he pressed a buzzer around his neck. Don would dash down only to find that Harold had locked himself into his bungalow good and fast. Harold's front door had several bolts and chains across it, rendering the fact that Don was a key holder, useless. The ambulance men then had to be called and they got very adept at breaking in through Harold's kitchen window. Thankfully, he was as tough as old boots, and never came to any harm.

But one sunny Saturday afternoon, we went down to Brixham breakwater with nine-year-old Tim to do a bit of fishing, and we took Harold with us to give him a nice day out.

On the bustling Breakwater which was buzzing with dog walkers and people out enjoying the fresh sea air, Don and Tim got their fishing rods baited up. Meanwhile, Harold sat on a bench and enjoyed a flask of tea and a biscuit.

Then Tim got a bite on his line.

Great excitement ensued as he reeled in the fish—a tiny wrasse.

Harold was over the moon and swanned off to get a bucket of water to keep the fish in.

'Don't throw it back in the sea yet, I'll fetch yer some water, lad,' he enthused.

So off he waddled down the slipway, bucket in hand. The tide was going out, and the slipway was covered in green, slimy algae—a slippery slope for sure.

But this did not deter Harold, who was determined to get a bucket of water.

You can guess what happened next.

Harold, a portly 92-year-old, gracefully slipped on the slipway feet first into the harbour and floated into the sea like a giant blow-up doll.

'Man overboard! Man overboard!' Don yelled, his voice frantic with panic, hoping to rouse the attention of passers-by and rustle up some help.

But no one took a scrap of notice.

'Help! Help!' Don bellowed, persisting. 'Help! Help! Man overboard!'

I dashed down the breakwater to the RNLI station to see if there was anyone there that could help; Harold had only just gone and slipped right in front of the RNLI rescue launch. But it was closed.

Tim, curious, calm and as cool as a cucumber, abandoned his fishing rod and followed me down just as some fishermen responded to Don's cries, and came to the rescue. They managed to drag Harold up the slipway like a beached whale. His clothes were sopping wet, and all he wanted to do was to get home, get changed and have a cup of tea.

But some bright spark had called an ambulance, which promptly arrived and took Harold off to the local hospital where they got him undressed, dried, checked over, and eventually sent him home after I'd collected some clean clothes for him. He was not a happy bunny.

I got handed a black bin liner with his sodden sea-soaked clothes inside to take home and wash. My washing machine was never the same again. The stench of slimy seawater lingered for weeks, permeating all our clothes. In the end, we had to buy a new one.

At least Tim had a story to tell his mates at school. They all thought his granddad was brill.

95. MORE CORNISH CAPERS

It's a gloriously hot day in July 2023, and we're visiting the delightful fishing village of Polperro. We join some people sitting on benches overlooking the inlet as we quaff our half-pints of Korev[1] Cornish lager.

There's a young guy eating lunch out of a takeaway container using his plastic driving licence card to shovel it into his mouth.

'Well, I think I've seen everything now,' I remark to him, laughing.

'It's the only way to eat a seafood salad when you've trodden on your plastic fork,' he informs me with a smile.

Don strikes up a conversation with all types of people wherever we go, and it inevitably leads him to tell people about some of the books I've written which I always find rather embarrassing.

'He's my agent,' I remark with a smile, giving a nod towards Don in an attempt to avert my discomfiture. Today is no exception, as he does his sales pitch to his captive audience seated on the bench.

'My wife's a best-selling Amazon author, you know,' he gloats, bringing up my book on his iPhone and showing everyone.

'Yes,' I concur, 'but only in a *very* obscure category on Amazon, tax law!' I assert to qualify his comment, which always gets a bit of a laugh.

'My wife's written a book about me, too. I used to be a busker, and it's called…' and off he goes chattering and nattering to his listeners who seem to find him amusing, I must say, to the point where one of the ladies asks to have a selfie with us.

'I've got a photo with the author now,' she says.

I then enjoy an invigorating swim in the tiny harbour at Polperro, which is deep and buoyant. I find I can float with ease —all fours stretched out. Normally I sink.

Then, dressed and refreshed, I buy my very first *Affogato* from a charming kiosk on the picturesque quay. The skilled barista pours a steaming cup of top-notch black coffee over a scoop of delectable Cornish ice cream, creating a heavenly fusion of flavours. The velvety smoothness of the ice cream mingles with the bold and robust essence of the coffee, making each spoonful an exquisite sensation. It's hard to believe how just two simple ingredients taste so divine.

We then travel on to Looe for fish and chips, which we eat overlooking the river in the evening sun. The fish is dreadfully overcooked. The fryer has murdered it, rendering it dry and tasteless, and the batter is slightly burnt. It's such a disappointing end to a fabulous day. The meal wasn't cheap either, at nearly £30 for two haddock and chips. I wish we'd had a Cornish pasty instead, but we'd been looking forward to eating some locally caught fresh fish.

We then head back to our van by crossing over the bridge to West Looe and pass diners sitting outside on the terrace of a posh restaurant at Hannafore. We're envious of the delicious meals they're tucking into, accompanied by large glasses of chilled white wine.

'Well, at least someone's enjoying some nice food,' I observe gloomily, feeling low-spirited with the taste of burnt batter still in the back of my throat.

'Lucky bastards,' says Don.

We laugh out loud at the incongruity of Don's language about the people innocently enjoying their evening repasts. His tongue-in-cheek comment helps to lighten our mood. *Maybe we'll dine there one day and be lucky bastards, too.*

¹ *A Cornish lager brewed at St Austell Brewery*

96. PAIGNTON

Working as a pianist at various hotels, I discovered that a "cosy winter break" is an affordable way to enjoy a short holiday in the UK in the dead of winter, and added to that, making a booking for early January will almost certainly guarantee a free room upgrade as the hotel is virtually empty. No one wants to go on holiday during the first week of January.

But we do.

So I search local hotel deals for dinner, bed and breakfast and we get a four-night winter break for £250 each. Added to this, we won't have a long drive and we'll turn our heating off—quids in. Holidays in some British hotels are now great value for money compared to what they were in the 1990s.

We arrive at the hotel in Paignton after a short five-mile drive from our home. Bliss.

Don transfers from the driver's seat into his electric wheelchair and then it all goes downhill.

First, he takes with him all the loose wires protruding from the two cigarette lighter plugs, which have somehow wrapped around his foot. There are wires from the dormant sat nav, wires from a mobile phone charger, and wires from a defunct dash cam, along with a strap from his holdall bag.

I untangle everything.

Then my foot gets caught in the handle of a black plastic bag, which is swanning around the passenger seat just as Don's keyring hanging from his pocket gets caught around the seat belt and tears his leather jacket.

I should explain here that Don's key ring is a force to be reckoned with. It's actually a dog lead chain—long and heavy, and he's got a bunch of keys at BOTH ends of the dog lead.

Just as Don is about to get out of the van by positioning his wheelchair on the lift, the electric controller gets trapped between the lift and the passenger seat and throws a hissy fit as it's triggered into action prematurely. This causes the lift to get jammed because the front wheels of the wheelchair are wedged over the lip of the lift.

Everything is now jammed.

The wheelchair is stuck, the lift is stuck, and the controller is stuck.

Don has to get out of his wheelchair and stumble back into the driver's seat, and after much huffing and puffing, we get everything unstuck. We might as well have travelled for several hours the way we feel after all that. We're exhausted.

We unpack the van, and Don goes off with luggage piled high on his knees just as his wheelchair seat belt gets mangled in the wheels (a frequent occurrence), and his best Marks & Spencer Fedora hat blows off and lands in a large puddle.

Well, it would, wouldn't it?

It's ruined.

We're given the best room in the hotel with a marvellous sea view - a free upgrade - and are welcomed with a complimentary cream tea. We have a most wonderful time doing nothing much at all. It's such good value that we book another four nights in March as the "cosy winter break" offer is still on then.

My quarterly tax-free payment from my solar panels will fund the holiday. I bought the solar panels with some of the money my father left me, and it's one of the best investments I could have made. It's like getting a cheque from my dad every quarter. He'd be well pleased.

Come March, we're not so lucky with the room at the cheap price we paid. I was expecting this, particularly as there's a coach load of other guests staying. We would definitely be bottom of the pile for rooms.

The room that the hotel allocates to us is inaccessible for Don's electric wheelchair (though it would have been fine if he'd been in a manual wheelchair), so we're given another room right at the back of the hotel which isn't disabled-friendly at all. The hotel manager and one of his colleagues have to rearrange half the furniture so that Don can get his wheelchair around the bed and into the bathroom.

It's not a great room, but it will have to do.

I unpack everything, which includes a plethora of wires and chargers.

There's a charger for the wheelchair.

There are chargers for our laptops, iPhones and Don's iPad.

There are chargers for my hearing aids and my Kindle.

Then there's Don's electric heat pad. He likes the pad on his tummy if he feels a bit 'delicate' (as he puts it).

The room is a liability with all the chargers and wires and I always worry about overloading the electric plug. Our extension lead is at full pelt.

What if we start a fire?

The next day, Don wants to have a bath.

'The bathwater looks a bit of a funny colour to me Don,' I observe after I've filled the bath, which is wonderfully deep. The water has a green tinge to it. Don thinks it's fine, which surprises me as he's hot on such things, being extremely wary about picking up infections from even the smallest of health hazards. However, he's happy to go ahead, and he gets in easily enough and enjoys a relaxing soak for half an hour. But the bath is so deep that he can't get out. Added to that, his weight is now nearly 19 stone which adds to the difficulty. He struggles for a good 20 minutes, but he's like a beached whale.

He gets very hot and breathless trying to lever himself up over the rim of the deep bath. The paralysis in his legs causes them to have no vigour - they're ineffectual. He has a lot of upper-body strength, but it's proving useless in this situation.

I'm on the verge of proposing that we call for help when I suggest to Don he get on all fours and climb out that way.

It works.

I run a bath for myself straight after and the water is crystal clear. There was surely something dodgy about the water in Don's bath and I guessed that the room hadn't been used for many, many months, but I didn't mention it to Don who has collapsed into bed. The exertion of trying to get out of the bath has knocked him up.

I nip down to the bar for a glass of ice, then take it up to our room and pour myself a gin and tonic, which I sip as I read a book while Don amuses himself on his laptop.

We nibble some cocktail nuts.

'Where's my phone charger wire?' Don enquires. His mobile needs charging two or three times a day (I bet a thousand open tabs are lurking).

'It's definitely there. I put it in the plug with the USB holes in the extension lead.'

'Well, I can't see it.'

I investigate and can see the phone charger wire plugged in, so I trace it along with my fingers up under the bedclothes, which I pull back only to find the end of the wire wrapped around his big toe.

How on earth did it get there?

'If it can happen, it will,' observes Don, spouting a frequent mantra of ours.

Soon it's time to get ready for dinner, so I set about helping Don to get dressed. I find four nuts digging into his hip, and discovering he's been lying on a *pain au chocolat* that he'd kept from breakfast. It was not a pretty sight.

97. MALVERN

We find another bargain hotel break for retired civil servants at a hotel in Malvern. We're the only people in the large dining room because we like to eat early at 6 p.m. Our group is booked to dine at 7 p.m. and everyone else is upstairs in the bar, drinking an apéritif.

Our starters arrive - Brussels pâté for me and salmon mousse for Don. He looks at his mousse glumly as the waiter places it before him.

'It's out of a tin,' he whispers, passing judgment on its appearance (I'm not sure why he's whispering, as we're the only people in the restaurant).

'What makes you say that?'

'Look at the shape of the slice. It's out of a tin,' he murmurs in hushed tones, even though there's not a soul about.

'I don't think so, it's been set in a terrine mould and come out shaped like that,' I reassure him, but I can see he's got a thing about it. He eats it in silence and we enjoy the rest of our meal.

The next evening we are, once again, the only diners at 6 p.m. on the dot. Our pre-ordered starters arrive. Soup for Don, with a ham and pea terrine for me.

'The only salmon mousse I could find on Google was for cats,' states Don. '£20 for six tins. Shaped like that,' he says, pointing with his soup spoon to my ham and pea terrine, which is the same shape the salmon mousse was.

... ahh, so that's it. Don thinks the hotel gave him cat food.

I shake my head in disbelief.

'They wouldn't do that, Don.'

He purses his lips.

I can see he's not convinced.

The holiday is excellent value again, especially as it's in the middle of August when prices are normally inflated.

Don hires a Tramper at Malvern Hills Geopark, and we meet up with our friend Mike. We go right to the top of Great Malvern, where the views are spectacular. These Trampers are a fantastic boon for disabled people because they allow them to enjoy riding safely over rough terrain and steep gradients. For £10 a year, Don can hire one at country venues all over the UK.

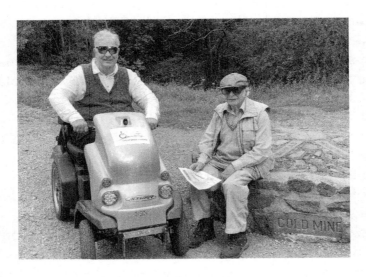

Don on the Tramper on Great Malvern
(and Mike sitting on a gold mine!)

98. STRATFORD

While we're in Malvern, we visit Stratford-upon-Avon, which is a favourite place of ours. I walk alongside Don's electric wheelchair down the River Avon and back, and we then head for the shops. It's quite a trek. Don, being in his wheelchair, doesn't feel the physical effects of walking long distances. I'm flagging somewhat—my sciatica is playing up and I'm whacked by the time we reach the shops. I'm on a mission to buy a long-line floral jacket to wear when I play the piano at the hotel. Don agrees it would look exceedingly classy.

'Follow me!' orders Don, waving his hand, and off he goes before I can object. He's going down a road which I just know will have no clothes shops whatsoever. I follow him, limping, trying hard to keep up with sciatica pain burning in my right hip and plantar fasciitis in my left foot. I'm like the walking wounded. But he's off down Windsor Street at top speed where there aren't any shops at all. There's everything but—there's a pub, a solicitor's, a cafe selling bubble tea, and a myriad of nondescript office buildings. It's a wild goose chase as we eventually come back full circle to the main shopping drag.

'Let's forget the jacket,' I pant. 'I'll have to stop and have a rest. I'm so hot. I could do with an ice-cold lager somewhere. I'm pooped,' I implore.

At a quaint pub alongside the tranquil River Avon, we relish the crisp taste of our refreshing drinks. We cool down, watching the ducks put their arses up in the air (as they do), creating a playful spectacle.

As I bask in the shade quaffing my half-pint, I reflect on the last time we'd visited Stratford back in 2012. Don was

265

into his busking and he'd packed his piano accordion. He was determined to do some busking on the streets of Stratford. After a bit of hassle with a policeman trying to find a "legal" place to busk, I helped him set up all his gear and made sure that Sammy, our Cavalier King Charles Spaniel, was comfortably sitting next to Don's wheelchair. Our dog seemed to enjoy being with Don while he played because everybody made a fuss of him (the dog that is, not Don).

The Olympics had just finished in London, and the Malaysian Olympic Team was visiting Stratford, sightseeing. They stopped to listen to Don playing for a while.

He fascinated them.

They even requested a song called "Streets of London" which Don willingly obliged them with. Not only that, Don made them all sing along to it, which they were pleased to do. And so it was that the Malaysian Olympic Team sang "Streets of London" on the streets of Stratford. How quirky is that?

They took lots of photographs of Don playing his accordion with Sam at his side. I guess he was quite a spectacle to the Malaysians. Maybe they don't have buskers in Malaysia? Or maybe it was Sam they liked. But whatever they warmed to, they presented Don with a Malaysian Olympic Team commemorative medal. Don was delighted with it, but the spin he put on this story to friends and relatives, you'd think they'd presented him with a real Olympic Gold Medal.

99. BOURNEMOUTH

'Can I have a screwdriver please, darling?' asks Don.

I'm helping Don to repair his handcycle before we go off to Bournemouth for a cheap 4-night stay there. Fixing the cycle is a two-person job, and Don needs me to hold his cycle steady while he works on it.

I get the screwdriver and hand it to him.

'Not that sort. I need a pod screwdriver.'

I roll my eyes and toddle off back to the utility room to get a "pod" screwdriver. Now, there is no such thing as a "pod" screwdriver, but Don does not know this. What he actually means is a "Phillips" screwdriver, but I've got used to his way with words. I get the "pod" screwdriver.

Two minutes later, there's another request.

'I need a bradawl.'

I get the bradawl.

'Can you get me some pliers, please?'

I get some pliers with a sigh and hand them to Don.

'No, not that sort. I need the pliers with a small pointy end.' I go back and search out the required tool.

Less than 30 seconds later, another request.

'Have you got a small hammer?'

'Crikey Don, this is getting ridiculous! Why don't you just tell me all the things you need before we start? It's getting like that Four Candles scene out of The Two Ronnies,' I quip. 'A bit of forward-thinking would help.' I moan as I experience empathy with Ronnie Corbett.

We get the job done.

Don is well pleased, as it means he can take his handcycle on holiday and enjoy a ride up and down the superb seafront at Bournemouth.

It's another cheap holiday at a hotel that does a special rate for retired civil servants. The group puts on these holidays all over the country at hotels where they get special deals.

As we pull up at the hotel, my heart sinks when I discover that we have to park Primrose (our van, which has a high roof) quite a long way from the hotel reception. There's a height restriction for parking close to the hotel, which means we can't drive Primrose under the car park roof.

'Drat! It'll take me ages to get all our luggage into our room,' I whinge.

'You worry too much, darling. They'll have one of those bellboy trolley thingies. Ask them for one, and we'll get all the luggage into the room in one go.'

To my relief, the hotel does indeed have a bellboy trolley (not every hotel does) and we pile everything onto it—two large suitcases, a large bag containing medical accoutrements that Don needs, several bags, Don's laptop bag, and my beloved soft pillow. Off I go, pulling it behind me over the uneven, pot-holed surface of the car park, which badly needs new tarmac.

Don whizzes by in his wheelchair just as the front wheel of the bellboy breaks off and all the luggage sprawls across the car park.

I am mortified.

Don swiftly fetches two porters to assist us, and with their amazing help, we're soon in our room, luggage and all. It's a twin-bedded affair with a large accessible bathroom (though I won't mention the issues I have with the teeny sink and the pathetic mixer tap that only spews out lukewarm water whichever way it's turned).

The beds are phenomenal, however, as they are both electric and we can position them however we want using a controller attached to them. Apart from Don falling in between the two beds one night (not to be recommended if you're 19 stone), it's a comfortable room although like most accessible rooms it's at the back of the hotel with a grim view of the rubbish bins. Still, we only sleep there.

The hotel is exceptional in catering for disabled people, including an amazing portable hoist by the outdoor heated swimming pool.

Don is determined to try out this poolside extravaganza, so with an audience of onlookers all enjoying an afternoon drink by the pool in the scorching April sunshine, the hotel manager positions Don ready to lower him into the water on this amazing device. It's a very vocal affair with many "whoops" and "ohs" from Don as the water reaches his nether regions, but he gets a round of applause from everyone once he's in. It's rather entertaining to watch.

A lot of these English hotels have live entertainment, and we often enjoy a dance after dinner. Our rhythmic movements delight everyone and we're straight in as soon as the music starts, with Don gliding in his wheelchair while I whirl and twirl around him. Then we stop moving and face each other, mirroring each other's movements as we twirl our fists around each other, and pump the air up and down like John Travolta. Occasionally other women come and dance with him too as they find it a fresh experience - it releases their inner dancer. It seems to make people feel good that someone with a disability can have a great time on the dance floor and is happy to enjoy themselves in front of them. Don is elated when people comment on how much they appreciate watching him "wheelchair dance".

'Did you know your husband can say he's danced with a hooker!' says one lady who'd joined in dancing with Don. 'My name's Audrey Hooker you see!'

The food is good, though I couldn't help but notice that the age of the waiting staff is around 18. There's a great chasm of years between waiting staff and guests. We're like a different species.

Don, as usual, chats with the young waiting staff and he discovers that not all of them are paid anything at all. One of the young waiters tells us he does it for nothing once a week as "work experience".

This shocks us.

We also feel rather guilty.

I deeply deplore such exploitation. *So that's why the holiday is so cheap?*

We would have preferred to pay a little extra so that all the young waiting staff could receive at least a minimum wage.

Now, what do you do when you inadvertently eat the after-dinner mint of the person you're sitting next to as well as your own?

Don eats the *Elizabeth Shaw* chocolate mint off his saucer to his right while he's waiting for his starter. Then, as coffee is served after our meal, he absent-mindedly helps himself to the mint off the saucer of the lady sitting next to him on his left as he natters away to her.

She doesn't notice.

But I do.

I tick him off.

She sees the funny side, and Don makes a joke of it.

I give her my chocolate instead.

We enjoyed a pleasant holiday with no hiccups and Don's handcycle repair thrilled him as he cycled up and down the gorgeous "golden mile" of Bournemouth seafront.

It's our last evening and I stroll down the hill to meet Don after his ride, just as dusk is falling. We breathe in the sea air and watch the young people having fun before making our way back to the hotel together.

'Follow me!' commands Don as he zips up the main road. It's strange, but for some reason, I don't want to go along the main road. I want to take the pedestrian footpath instead, where the goats feed off the scrub along the hillside. But Don is off before I can object.

His handcycle is power-assisted, enabling him to reach a fair speed, ascending hills effortlessly. I can't keep up with him.

He disappears around a bend and I hear him cry out. Something is wrong.

100. PLEASE PARK CAREFULLY

I quicken my pace to a run to catch him up.

I find Don lying on his left side.

His handcycle has tipped over. A crowd has already gathered around him and they're trying to help him up (no mean feat, as he's almost 19 stone). One lady takes charge and tells several young men how to go about it, and I'm so grateful for their help. I could never have got him up back into the handcycle by myself. Don is badly shaken, but once he's sitting upright back on the cycle, he feels better. We thank everyone and make it back to the hotel, which isn't far away.

Don explains the reason he'd overturned was because a car was parked incorrectly and this caused him to swerve, forcing his handcycle to go down a kerb and tip over.

Cars parked incorrectly are a common misdemeanour by drivers. A wheelchair needs space on pavements, and cars parked over the kerb force wheelchair users onto the road.

Don's safety helmet had protected his head, but his left shoulder had taken the brunt of the fall. Despite his age of 77, his bones are strong and there's no damage either to him or, miraculously, to his handcycle.

However, the shock kicks in once we're back in our room and it causes Don to have a very upset tummy that night. It was not a nice way to end the holiday.

101. WARNER LEISURE HOTELS

We get a discount offered at Warner Leisure Hotels through the retired civil service group we belong to and we decide to give it a whirl. I never thought I'd sample one of these holidays, but some of them are good value for money.

The venue we chose used to be a castle in times gone by, and the long corridors leading to all the rooms resemble those of a cruise liner. These adult-only holidays are especially suitable for people with mobility problems—Don can get his wheelchair virtually everywhere.

We arrive late on our first evening because of my work commitments, and as we enter the restaurant, there's a sea of grey hair and four walking aids lined up against the wall.

Once again, I notice a significant age gap between the waiting staff and the guests. The waiters are around 18, while the guests are around 80—many of whom have health and mobility issues and use scooters, walkers, and other aids. The place resembles a care home with all the Zimmer frames scattered around. At 63 years old, I must be one of the youngest guests there.

And yet, I'm loving seeing all these senior citizens having a great time in the last lap of life, sipping cocktails, gin and tonics, large glasses of wine and spending their pensions on leisure and pleasure.

I'd witnessed similar scenes over the years at the hotel where I play the piano during dinner, especially during "Turkey and Tinsel" time. The pensioners give it some welly and have a ball.

The atmosphere is buzzing, full of loud laughter and chatter, blowing party horns and letting off balloons which fart their way around the restaurant (sometimes landing on me or the piano).

"For the living know that they will die" is a phrase that comes to my mind when I'm in such places, and I admire these people as they keep going and resist the care homes.

But then, out of the blue, a derogatory phrase involuntarily pops into my head about these elderly guests. It's a phrase once used by a young Baptist pastor in Brixham in one of his Facebook status updates, where he refers to the ageing population of Brixham wandering around the town as "coffin dodgers".

'Look at all us coffin dodgers,' I say to Don as we assemble in the theatre to watch the show after dinner. Don knows exactly where I got the phrase from and remembers it well.

'That little pipsqueak knows nothing. He might have been to Bible college, but he should know better than to make short-sighted comments like that!' he quips back. 'He'll be a coffin-dodger himself one day.'

The entertainment laid on at Warner Leisure is also cruise-ship-like in that it's nightly, with variety shows, singers and discos, comedians and magicians. On our first night there, it's a very good comedian (a rare treat for us) and I enjoy seeing people in their late 80s and early 90s laughing until the tears run down their faces. It's like a shot in the arm to see them dodging the coffins with such mirth and merriment. It's an uplifting experience.

We just hope that all the junior staff are being paid and aren't doing it for free as "work experience". We notice how they all work so hard and it's relentless for them, preparing the tables, serving, clearing away, and then doing it all again.

There's an indoor pool with a hoist and Don decides he'd like a swim, so we get changed in our room and off we go to the spa. The hoist is nifty, and two members of staff lower Don safely into the pool, once again to the accompaniment of his many "whoops" and "ohs" as the lukewarm water gets higher and higher up his body, but once he's in he acclimatises.

But then, without warning, Don gets into trouble.

102. DRAMA IN THE POOL

Don keeps falling backwards and his head goes underwater.

It's unclear why this is so because he's a fairly good swimmer having a lot of upper body strength, but he's lost his balance and is taking in water.

In a flash, the two attendants, Tash and Sam, are right there by the pool. Tash encourages Don to come towards the edge, but try as he might, he keeps falling backwards, swallowing water.

Tash jumps in fully clothed and tries to calm him and get him upright, but it's not working. His head keeps submerging, and he's gulping.

'Hug me!' demands Tash, in an effort to get Don upright in the water.

'Oooh, I was hoping you'd say that, Tash,' says Don, as he puts his arms around her neck.

We all laugh.

But her quick thinking works, and Don is suddenly upright and stable.

In all seriousness, hugging Tash was indeed the best way to get Don vertical and to the edge of the pool, where they get him out on the hoist. She is good at her job.

Undeterred, we go back the next day for another swim. But Don has been banned from swimming. We play ping-pong instead—though it was more ping than pong with my poor hand-to-eye coordination. As usual, I end up being the ping-pong ball picker-upper.

103. TORQUAY

We discovered local hotels have some excellent offers out of season, so we booked a cheap four-night break at a hotel in Torquay. Another quarterly cheque from my solar panels funds the holiday. My Dad would be over the moon.

It's a win-win: we don't have to buy any food, we turn off the heating, and it's only ten miles away. Quids in.

We arrive and unload.

'Don!' I call after him as he swans off toward the lift. 'The corner of your coat is getting mangled in your wheels!'

Don's long winter coat frequently gets ripped in this manner.

'No worries, Wendy'll fix it,' Don calls back.

Wendy is a long-time friend of ours and a superb needlewoman (unlike me), and she's forever mending Don's wheelchair-wrecked clothing, amongst other things.

We get settled into a pleasant room with a magnificent sea view and a complimentary cream tea—a free upgrade, which we are very grateful for.

At dinner, the restaurant is already almost full as we queue up to be shown to our table. I can't help noticing that, as usual, the hotel is packed with pensioners. Once again, I must be one of the youngest guests there at the age of 63.

I conclude pensioners keep all the hotels in the UK running and in business. They're the ones with no mortgages; they're the ones with time on their hands; they're the ones knowing time is short. Without the pensioners, there'd be no guests, and no guests mean no jobs for the young waiting staff. And no jobs for the staff would mean no pensions for the pensioners as the taxes the staff pay help to fund the State Pension. The old saying "money makes the world go around" comes to mind.

Don also notices the age of the guests. It's becoming a habit.

'Do you realise that there must be almost 3000 years of life experience in this dining room?' observes Don, as he counts the number of mature guests - around 45 people at an average age of 70.

'I hadn't thought of it like that, but yes, you're right.'

Don chats to our delightful waiter, Charmelo, who tells us that his mother gave him his unusual name because he was born in March, but his mother reversed "March" to "Charm" and then added the "elo" at the end.

We love it.

He's Charmelo by name and charming by nature and we enjoy a friendly exchange, telling us he's from the Philippines. Charmelo is poised with pen and pad in hand, ready to take our order.

Now, although Don claims he is a "vegan" he only identifies as one when he fancies it because he regularly eats eggs and fish. And occasionally chicken. And turkey. Tonight, fish is on the menu, but it's a fish that Don isn't familiar with.

'Tell me about the hake Charmelo,' asks Don, looking up expectantly, 'is it a bottom-feeder?'

Words cannot describe the look on Charmelo's face. Only an emoticon can sum it up:

'Don!' I object swiftly. 'Charmelo won't know the answer to that question! You'll have to google it.'

'I haven't got my phone.'

I get my phone, google "hake" and hand it to Don.

'You really needn't be worried about such things,' I reassure him, shaking my head.

'But bottom feeders eat up all the muck off the ocean floor,' he fires back.

'But you ate a crab sandwich in Looe a few months ago, and crabs are bottom-feeding crustaceans,' I rationalise, as poor Charmelo is still standing there with his pad in hand.

Don gives up the googling.

'OK, I'll have the mushroom soup to start and the hake for main. Thank you, Charmelo.'

Goodness knows what Charmelo made of our conversation about the hake, but the next evening at dinner, I noticed he was serving people at the opposite end of the restaurant!

We have a delightful break overall, apart from when Don gets stuck in the tiny lift, which went down to the basement of its own accord. His claustrophobia almost kicked in just as the engineers rescued him. And then when I'm helping Don to pull his trousers down, his legs collapse under him, as all 19 stone crushes my right hand against the wheelchair, causing agonising pain. Good job I didn't break any bones. I have to go to work and play the piano during dinner later that week.

104. FATHER AND SON TRIPS

BANG!!

I rush into the dining room where the bang comes from. Don is sitting in his wheelchair as white as a sheet at the dining table where he's sorting out his fishing tackle. He put a battery on charge for his rechargeable torch and it exploded. Not only has the explosion caused a scare, but it's also made a terrible mess - part of the wall is black, half of the radiator is black, several floor tiles are black and the battery and the charger are now defunct. Oh, and the wires are singed.

'It could have caused a fire!' I observe with alarm, stating the obvious. 'How did that happen?'

'It was a cheap one I bought off Amazon,' Don admits, looking down at it with disgust. 'I'm not sure why it exploded.'

He's getting ready to go on a fishing trip with Tim (who has now 'flown the nest' and works as a refrigeration and air conditioning engineer). They're off to fish at *Le Val Doré* Lakes in France. Tim takes over the role of carer on these trips (minus the bed baths), and apart from a flat battery in Primrose because Don used his wheelchair lift several times a day for a week without turning on the engine, they have a great time catching many fish.

Meanwhile, back in Brixham, Don's rechargeable torch is redundant and stays with me at home as I clean up the mess from the explosion. Living with a wheelchair user means that I've learnt not to be house-proud. Our property suffers many dilapidations from knocks and bashes as the wheelchair makes its mark on our decor. The woodwork is scuffed all around the skirting, three doors have gaping holes in them, a sliding mirrored door is cracked, and in the hall, there are parts where the wallpaper has been scraped off. It is what it is.

Don and Tim have not only fished at *Val Doré* in France but have also kept tight lines at Todber Manor in Dorset, catching giant ugly catfish in the middle of the night. A posse of Tim's friends join in the fishing fest, and Don enjoys cooking meals for the lads by the lakeside.

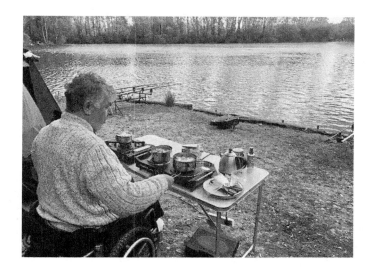

Don the chef—eat your heart out Jamie Oliver!

As well as fishing, they also share a keen enjoyment of cycling evidenced by their cycle trail adventures along the Danube and the Rhone. I never join them on these escapades because I cannot ride a bike. My balance is poor and I fall off.

On Don's 78th birthday, they plan their next cycle trip—a ride from Bristol Bridge to London Bridge. It will take them three days, and I will be driving the van to three hotels along the way for overnight stays.

This plan unfolds as we sit in a posh fine-dining restaurant in Totnes. But it comes to an abrupt halt when Tim struggles to stifle his laughter at the sight of Don dabbing his macaroon into the chocolate "Happy Birthday" message, resembling someone savouring brown sauce with a slice of bread. The sight of it sends Tim into a fit of laughter, his shoulders shaking, the atmosphere vibrating with amusement. Well, I guess you can't let any delectable chocolate sauce escape, can you?

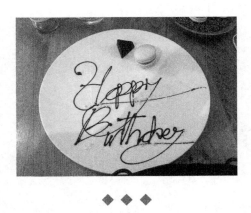

◆ ◆ ◆

While Don and Tim are away on their travels, I often take myself off to enjoy a trip on my own, usually a Cornish-fest where I explore as many Cornish fishing villages as possible. Villages such as Port Isaac, St. Ives, Polperro, Fowey, and Porthleven. It means I can do things and stay at places where accessibility is not an issue.

So, while Don and Tim are off to France, I decide to visit Mevagissey and then go on to the tiny fishing hamlet of Portloe. What could possibly go wrong?

105. MORE TRAVELS WITHOUT DON

Mevagissey is blocked off.

"Road Ahead Closed," the sign says.

I ignore it.

All the other motorists are ignoring it too and there are no "diversion" signs, so we just keep going.

This happens twice more.

We admit defeat when we see the workmen and their equipment up ahead. Yes, the road REALLY IS closed ...*of all the days to pick to come to Mevagissey.*

Not to be foiled, I find a different route around to Mevagissey, an extra 13 miles through very narrow Cornish lanes, but it is worth it.

I enjoy a marvellous lunch of fresh scallops followed by a coastal boat trip before heading onwards to Portloe 12 miles further to the West. I've booked into the charming Lugger Hotel (built in 1701 as an inn for bootleggers of French brandy, no less).

I love driving down narrow Cornish lanes where mossy grass is spouting in the middle and the hedges are almost eight feet high.

As I approach the hamlet of Portloe, the road widens, and I pass a picturesque cottage which has sexy underwear hanging on the line in the front garden, including a lacy red thong.

Well, I didn't see that coming.

I have to smile.

It's not the sort of thing one imagines to find in a Cornish fishing hamlet, is it? I just have to stop and take a photo. I mean, who'd have thought it?

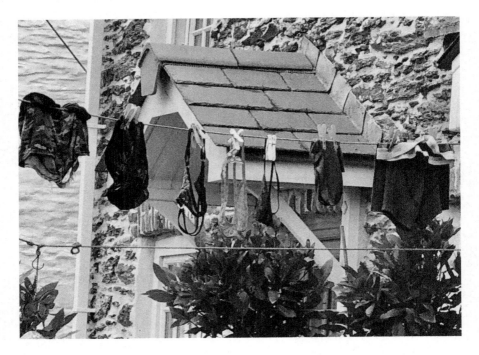

My sat nav informs me I have just 175 yards (yes, yards) to reach the Lugger Hotel, which sits right on the beach at Portloe.

Just before I turn left onto the bijou beach, my jaw drops.

106. RIGHT
SAID FRED

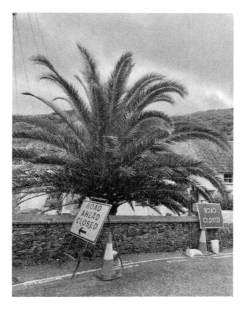

"Road Ahead Closed," says the sign.

What again? With just 175 yards to go?

What are the chances of two Cornish fishing villages having roads blocked off on the same day? Mevagissey, I could understand. It's a large town.

But Portloe?

There are no workmen this time and there's not a soul around, so I ignore the sign and drive perilously over a hole in the road. I need to get to the car park at The Lugger Hotel to check in and unpack. The hotel is inaccessible for wheelchair users due to its age, so for me, this is a fresh experience to stay in such a quaint venue, and I relish all the nooks and crannies of its quirky design.

It has crossed my mind a few times that maybe I'm a bit of a jinx when we travel because every time Don and Tim go away together, it all seems hunky-dory for them where nothing goes wrong.

I experience three blissful days in Portloe exploring various delightful local villages. The hotel's food, sourced fresh and local, satisfies the soul. Yet, it is the alluring morning and evening "blue hour" phenomenon at twilight that truly captures my heart. Rising early, I am greeted by the gentle hues of the morning blue hour, while later on, I indulge in the lingering tranquillity of the evening blue hour. The sun's blue rays gracefully caress the hotel's white façade, enveloping it in an aura of serenity and peace. This ethereal sensation remains with me, permeating my senses throughout the day and night.

On my way home I decide to stop off at Fowey, but two more "Road Ahead Closed" signs blight my trip. Then the "diversion" signs disappear.

I get hopelessly lost.

After much faffing around, I make it into Fowey, with my newly washed car splattered in mud and muck from the narrow Cornish roads churned up by the farmers' tractors. Apart from getting shat upon by a seagull, I have a lovely time mooching through the quirky shops.

It's good to be going home (isn't it always?) and the A38 is clear.

I make fast progress.

I'm on the home straight now. No more "Road Ahead Closed" signs.

I'll be home within the hour. It's plain sailing all the way, isn't it?

107. ROAD CLOSED

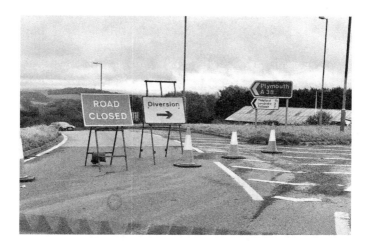

There it is again on the A38. "Road Closed".

For some strange reason, I'm not at all surprised. It's almost as if I'm expecting it.

I won't bore you with all the trouble this roadblock caused, not only me, but many other motorists. Oh, and the "diversion" sign was useless as it just sent the driver around and around the roundabout. It didn't divert us anywhere.

What should have been an hour's drive home ended up being two and a half hours slog through Callington to get to Saltash because of all the intricate waterways around Plymouth.

I'm so vexed by all the hassle that I do something I've never done in my life before when I finally reach Plymouth - I stop off at McDonald's and buy myself a fish burger with fries and coke, the lot.

Oddly enough, it did help to soothe the soul a bit.

◆ ◆ ◆

But back to Tim and Don and their joint adventures. When they travel together, Tim helps with some of Don's caring needs. Tim has helped not only on these holidays but also as he grew up. When he was 12, he wrote a poem about it.

Two Are Better Than One
by Tim the Carer

My Dad's in a wheelchair because he's disabled.
As one of his carers, I try to make him enabled.
I can fetch the cordless phone,
Without giving a groan.
I also open the door,
But there's also so much more.
I can make him smile when he feels low,
It's all part of being a carer, you know.
We work together as a team,
It's not as easy as it might seem.

I've washed my Dad's hair,
While he sits in his chair,
I've given him a shampoo,
And I've blow-dried it too!
(I've even made sure he can get to the loo!)

It can be quite tiring, pushing the chair
Even if we don't aim to take off in the air.
My Dad helps me too,
When I've homework to do -
Two are better than one,
And much better than none!

I can't remember all that I do,
Just being there, and making a stew,

These are some of the things, to name but two.

But I must finish now,
Because there's lots more to do.
I hear my Dad calling,
I'm off, just in case he's falling.
Being a carer is being a pair,
It's all about really showing you care.

108. CARERS

Tim has always been very helpful and has been happy to share some of the caring duties with me over the years, and also now as an adult. He's an air conditioning and refrigeration engineer and his engineering skills come in extremely handy when Don's bike or wheelchair needs maintenance or repair.

The poem Tim wrote all those years ago was a light-hearted take on his helping hand and he genuinely enjoyed helping his Dad when he could, but I was surprised to learn that in the UK, there are around 800,000 child carers (some as young as five) who help to look after a family member. As an adult carer, I know only too well how depleting and stressful it can be at times, so it must be hard for a child to take on the sole responsibility of being a carer.

When Don and Tim travel together, it gives me time and space to experience travel alone, offering me a different perspective and the gift to explore places requiring mobility. Nothing special—just simple things, such as enjoying a meal upstairs on the balcony of the Red Lion pub overlooking the harbour in Port Isaac, which is one of my favourite places in all the world (and now a famous place since it featured in the TV series *Doc Martin* and the *Fisherman's Friends* movie). A wheelchair user can't experience this because of the pub's quaint design. Many old buildings are not wheelchair accessible, and this will always be the case in such structures.

When Don returns from his travels with Tim, he's always on a high, talking about all the great things they've experienced, filling me in on all the good times.

One year, he's invited to give a charity talk at Dart Sailability about their two charity cycle rides and I look forward to hearing Don's talk. This will be the first time I've heard about the trips in any detail.

It's not what I'm expecting at all.

PART NINE - FATHER AND SON TRIP

*The Beautiful Blue Danube
Charity Bike Ride*

109. THE TRAIL

My little theory that everything is hunky-dory on their trips gets blown apart. As I sit and listen to Don and watch his PowerPoint presentation, I learn the truth.

Well, well, well. I had no idea!

Here is their story.

Cue "The Blue Danube" music.

A father and son cycle trip abroad has become a passion. Don researches some cycle trails and is drawn to the River Danube, which stretches 1780 miles from its source in Germany to the Black Sea, where there's the enchanting Danube Cycle Trail, Europe's renowned cycling route from Passau to Vienna.

Spanning some 220 miles, this picturesque trail unveils a serene journey alongside the River Danube, cascading 200 feet between Passau and Vienna.

The well-maintained path guides cyclists through a tapestry of spectacular landscapes, adorned with resplendent palaces, hilltop castles, tranquil monasteries, and quaint, delightful villages.

Each pedal stroke, Don learns, is a symphony of beautiful sights and scents. What's not to like about this idyllic haven where nature and history blend?

So, in September 2017, Don and Tim began their journey, raising money for the charity PHAB—an organisation which inspires and supports disabled and non-disabled children alike.

They set off from Brixham in Primrose for the car ferry at Dover. The 1000-mile drive is a two-day adventure filled with breathtaking landscapes and the hum of the open road.

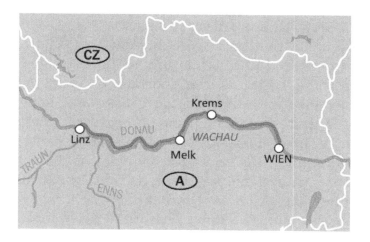

Exhausted yet exhilarated, they arrive in Linz - their base camp for three nights - just in time to savour a delicious dinner at the campsite restaurant. The aroma of freshly cooked food wafts through the air, enticing their growling stomachs. Then, with their hunger satisfied, a good night's sleep comes easily to them.

Early next morning, they scoff a hearty breakfast and catch the train to Passau in Germany, where they begin their ride— Don with his handcycle, Tim on his bike.

After cycling 21 miles back towards Linz in Austria, where their base camp is, they reach the *Schlögener Schlinge* (Schlongen Bend), which gives a stunning view of the curve in the River Danube as it snakes into a 180-degree turn. A cycle ferry carries them to the other side where there's a pleasant hotel overlooking the Danube—a perfect place for lunch.

Determined to try the tantalising local cuisine, Tim enthusiastically chooses the world-famous *wiener schnitzel*, Austria's national dish. Don opts for the flavourful Austrian goulash. The exotic fusion of aromas stimulates their senses. This is just the kind of experience they were hoping for.

It's also their first encounter with the *Radler* drink, a

delightful concoction that leaves a lasting impression on them. Derived from the German word for cyclist - *Radfahrer* - the name perfectly embodies its origins.

Legend has it that on a scorching day in 1922, a massive group of cyclists, some estimating 3000, descended upon a Bavarian pub. Aghast at the shortage of beer, the quick-thinking owner mixed equal parts beer and lemon soda, birthing a refreshing, low-alcohol beverage named after the cyclists themselves—*Radler*. Today, over a century later, travellers can find this beloved drink being sold all along the picturesque Danube, inviting them to savour its zestful charm.

Reaching the *Schlogen* bend, an engaging wheelchair-accessible museum welcomes visitors to delve into the rich history of the Roman fortifications. The museum, nestled amidst the scenic surroundings, offers a sensory feast for curious minds. But alas, Don and Tim have no time to sample such sights—they press on.

As they breeze along the trail towards Linz, soaking up the natural beauty all around them, they cycle through a wooded area. Don is out in front, giving it some welly with his power-assisted battery. A train track crisscrosses the cycle trail, and Don picks up even more speed to bounce over it, as cyclists do.

But his front wheel gets jammed on the track, almost throwing him out of his wheelchair.

Then he hears a train coming around the bend...

110. TIM TO THE RESCUE

From out of nowhere, Tim is there right by his side, having caught him up fast.

In seconds, with adrenaline coursing through his veins, Tim pushes Don, his handcycle and his wheelchair, over the train track.

Just in time.

The jaunty train whistle sounds as it passes by.

Relief washes over them. Time for a *Radler*.

Next stop: Linz.

The allure of Linz lies in its magnificent baroque architecture, which stands as a testament to its grandeur, and in the streets, the aroma of freshly brewed coffee wafts through the air, enticing tourists to explore the city's renowned coffee shops.

One delicacy that Linz proudly claims as its own is the Linz Tart, a delectable pastry believed to be the first cake ever named after a place. Its mouthwatering recipe, passed down through generations, dates back to 1653.

Regrettably, Don and Tim have no spare time to relish sightseeing or savour any of the gifts that Linz has to offer. The day is drawing to a close and they have to head back to their base camp, Pichlingersee—a calm and picturesque oasis on the outskirts of the city, surrounded by lakes.

Following the well-signposted route, it's impossible to lose your way.

But Don and Tim find themselves disorientated. They are

lost.

111. PANIC ON THE DANUBE

As daylight fades, and with their mobile phones dead and in need of charging, they realise they have travelled a considerable distance, covering 66 miles.

Panic sets in as they become aware they are unfamiliar with the city's intricate web of streets. Consulting their maps, a glimmer of hope emerges: they can cross the Danube at the hydroelectric dams opposite their campsite.

Without hesitation, Tim surges ahead, his excitement palpable. Their gamble pays off, as they find themselves safely on the other side of the river. Relief washes over them for the second time that day as they make their way back to the campsite, grateful for the serendipitous discovery that's guided them home.

On the fourth day, they cycle from Linz to Melk, a distance of 66.9 miles, and the charming village of Grein seizes their attention. Its beauty is arresting, with delightful houses and streets adorned with a multitude of colourful blooms. Pedalling along, the sweet scent of blooming flowers encircles them, adding to the idyllic atmosphere. They discover Grein has a hidden gem—the oldest theatre in Austria, holding stories of centuries past and whispering secrets of performances and applause.

Continuing on their journey, they reach Melk, where the

stunning abbey awaits them. Perched atop a hill overlooking the majestic Danube River, its towering spires reach towards the skies. It's an active monastery where the abbey is home to several Benedictine monks. It's also a secondary school, bustling with students going about their daily activities, where the echoes of the past meet the promise of the future.

After a long and tiring six hours of cycling, their thirst grows unbearable. They yearn for a refreshing *Radler*—that magical beer and lemon soda mix, and their hopes rise as they spot a drink dispensing machine at the railway station.

But it's out of order, leaving them thirsty and disappointed.

In their moment of despair, a kind-hearted lady appears like an angel. She's noticed their predicament and immediately offers to buy them a drink at the hotel across the road. They accept her generous offer and learn that Miriam - now in her eighties - speaks excellent English. And so they chew the fat over their *Radlers* as the cool, citrusy taste quenches their thirst and rejuvenates their spirits.

It's time to get the train back to camp at Linz, but there's a problem.

The locomotive is not wheelchair accessible, and to top it all, the train manager, a tall and imposing figure, is disinterested in assisting them. He seems to relish in their helplessness and refuses to speak English, leaving them stranded at the station.

Now what are they to do?

112. AN UNLIKELY RESCUE

Their newfound friend Miriam appears by their side and surprises Don and Tim. Despite her age and petite stature, she possesses incredible determination and resilience. In a bold display, she confronts the train manager, passionately arguing with him in German. Animated gestures accompany her words as if she were painting a vivid picture with her hands.

This goes on for quite a while, and the train manager is having none of it.

But Miriam is having none of it either. In a battle of the wills, she wins. The train manager reluctantly relents. With his head hung low, he grudgingly fetches the manually operated wheelchair lift and assists Don onto the train. Miriam, their saviour, joins them for the rest of the journey, and her presence fills the air with joy. They can't help but smile, amazed at how one diminutive lady in her eighties has made such a monumental difference.

On the fifth day, they take a break from cycling and drive 104 miles to Tulln, a pleasant garden city nestled beside the Danube, just 25 miles away from Vienna. Don and Tim have planned to go fishing on the Danube, but the excessively high license fees make them change their mind.

Instead, they explore the area and soak up the sights and sounds of Tulln. It's a much-needed day of relaxation, taking in the picturesque views and enjoying the tranquillity of their surroundings. Tulln is to be their base camp for the next three nights, promising more exciting adventures in the days to come.

The following day, a sunny Thursday morning, they board the wheelchair-accessible train back to Melk. From Melk, they cycle to Tulln, where the breathtaking view of the Wachau Valley and the Danube River stretches out before them, its sparkling waters reflecting the golden rays of sunlight. They can almost smell the sweet scent of the apricot and grape orchards as they pass by the renowned farming region, famous for its high-quality wines and liquors.

The Wachau Valley, spanning 25 miles between Melk and Krems, holds a rich heritage.

It is such a stunning place that it earned a place on the UNESCO World Cultural Heritage Sites list in 2000, and the National Geographic Traveller Magazine recognised it as the Best Historic Destination in the World in 2008.

Despite its fame, words can't capture the beauty Don and Tim witness. Their photographs, though cherished, cannot do justice to the spectacular landscape.

Then their journey comes to an abrupt halt.

113. PIT STOP

Don has a puncture. Not a big issue, but inconvenient.

A pit stop is necessary to repair one of Don's wheelchair tyres, but soon enough, they are back on their way to Tulln.

As they continue their exploration, an interesting tale emerges. You've heard of the Lochness Monster—but have you heard of the beast of the Danube? (And no, that's not a reference to an unhelpful Austrian train manager!).

This beast was none other than the Danube salmon, a majestic creature capable of living up to 30 years and growing to the size of a man.

Sadly, because of the many hydroelectric dams obstructing their spawning grounds, the salmon had become an endangered species. But there was hope. Josef Fischer, a dedicated wine grower and angler, had taken it upon himself to breed thousands of salmon each year. His large tanks, nestled amidst the vines along the Danube, served as sanctuaries for these remarkable fish. Fischer, ironically named for his profession, admitted that his love for the salmon had led him to abstain from eating them for a decade.

As Don and Tim approach the end of the Wachau Valley, a bridge awaits them—the first in 25 miles.

So, how do cyclists ascend to the level of the bridge?

To their surprise, they have to navigate circular cycle tracks spiralling their way up. The dizzying ascent, around and around, is not an issue for Don or Tim, and they marvel at the ingenuity of the design.

Approaching Vienna, the landscape gradually transforms into a serene, flat expanse. Amidst this journey, Don tows his beloved piano accordion, eagerly anticipating his upcoming busking performance in the city that nurtured the talents of Beethoven and Strauss.

At last, they arrive in Vienna. Even the cycle lanes possess their own traffic lights, a testament to the city's commitment to organised transportation.

If you ever have the pleasure of visiting Vienna, be sure to indulge in the experience of its world-renowned coffee shops. Adorned with ornate interiors and artistic masterpieces, these establishments carry a rich history. Café Frauenhuber, the oldest coffeehouse in Vienna, once hosted the legendary performances of Mozart and Beethoven.

Even Dr. Sigmund Freud would treat his patients to a cup of coffee there before delving into their psychoanalysis sessions.

Don resists visiting these coffee shops because he's dedicated to busking, hoping to gather enough euros to fulfil his promise to buy a celebratory meal. Tim surprises him with a takeaway coffee before disappearing to explore the city's sights by himself and purchase some souvenirs. Diamonds aren't necessarily a "girl's best friend" you see. Chocolate is. Tim plans to buy some top-notch Austrian chocolate for his sweetheart, Becca.

Amidst the bustling city, one particular sound captures Don's attention—the resounding chimes of St. Stephen's Cathedral. With 22 powerful bells, the largest weighing over 22 tons, the cathedral holds the honour of housing Austria's largest bell and the second-largest swinging bell in all of Europe.

Vienna is landlocked, of course. Right? And yet it boasts seven beaches peppered with restaurants all along the banks of the Danube. There, one can recline in comfortable deck chairs, build sandcastles, bask in the sun, and visualise the Mediterranean while savouring a luscious meal. And that's just what Don and Tim do. Indulging in this delightful experience with the proceeds of the busking money, they relish the flavours of the food and the refreshing *Radlers* at the Tel Aviv beach on the Danube in Vienna.

All too soon, it's time to embark on the daunting 1000-mile journey back home. But first, they have to make their way to Vienna's bustling main railway station.

The Friday evening rush hour engulfs the station, as Viennese commuters eagerly seek solace for the weekend. Neither Tim nor Don understand German, which renders the departure and arrival boards unintelligible. What seems like hours pass as they search for an English speaker, only to realise they are at the wrong station.

With a population of over 2 million, Vienna boasts two major railway stations. Someone informs them that the quickest route between the two stations involves taking the underground. Their hearts sink at the very thought. Navigating underground trains during rush hour is an arduous task, even for non-disabled people.

Standing on the platform, they watch as trains zoom in, doors fling open, passengers spill out, and a fresh wave surges in with doors swiftly closing behind them—a disconcerting sight, to say the least.

How did they end up in this predicament?

How will they board the bustling tube train with Don's handcycle, trailer, piano accordion, wheelchair, Tim's bike, and his panniers filled to the brim with Vienna's finest chocolates for Becca?

What are they to do?

114. THE TALE OF TWO STATIONS

They must have appeared quite forlorn when, out of nowhere, a smartly dressed gentleman approaches them. Fluent in English, he selflessly offers his help. It's a miracle how they squeeze themselves onto the packed tube train, thanks to the kind-hearted stranger who recognised their plight and went out of his way to lend a hand. He refused any form of gratitude. One person truly has the power to transform a situation from failure to success.

At Tulln, a further problem awaits them—they're greeted with the news that the lift connecting the platform down to street level is out of order.

So now what are they to do?

There are three daunting flights of steep stairs descending to the street below. Panic sets in as Don and Tim exchange worried glances.

How are they going to navigate those treacherous steps with all their equipment?

115. HUMAN KINDNESS

Just when all hope seemed lost, two strapping young men appeared before them like magic.

'Can we help you?' they offer kindly.

Without hesitation, they effortlessly lift Don in his wheelchair, and with remarkable speed, descend the stairs. With his eyes squeezed shut, Don clings tightly to the wheelchair's armrests, his heart racing.

They make light work of bringing the remainder of their gear down to street level.

What a difference a little human kindness makes.

They safely pedal back to their base camp in Tulln. The experience of handcycling along the River Danube has been extraordinary, and Don yearns to do it again—next time allowing for a leisurely two-week journey. He would take more opportunities to immerse himself in the sights, sounds, and smells of the surroundings, ensuring a visit to a Vienna coffee shop.

This adventure with Tim is nothing short of epic. They both cherished every moment and the memories they created will undoubtedly endure a lifetime.

PART TEN - FATHER AND SON TRIP

*From the Source to the Sea -
River Rhone Charity Bike Ride*

116. JAMES BOND EAT YOUR HEART OUT

Cue the theme music to James Bond, and 2018 saw Don eagerly research and plan another long cycle trail. This time he's drawn to the breathtaking Rhone Valley bike ride from the source of the River Rhone, beginning at the majestic Furka Pass, right down to the Mediterranean Sea.

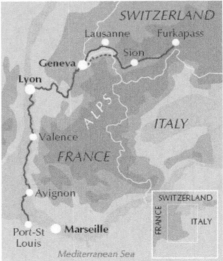

This time, their cause is to raise funds for the life-changing charity Compassion UK, which has already lifted over 86,000 children out of the clutches of poverty.

The journey to the Furka Pass is an arduous two-day drive, where Tim and Don share the driving duties. As dusk settles in on the first evening, they seek respite in the safety of a busy sprawling Autobahn service station, and they replenish their energy with a hearty breakfast the next morning.

On the second day of their expedition, after several hours of travelling, darkness descends as they ascend the Furka Pass to the place where they will spend the night.

A thick mist envelopes the van, reducing visibility to a mere haze. The fog lights, attempting to pierce through the mist, only reflect back at them.

Climbing the steep gradient, up, up, up they go, navigating countless, treacherous hairpin bends.

The mist morphs into a thick fog.

They drop speed and creep along in a slow-moving crawl, just about making out the occasional concrete pillars strategically placed to prevent motorists from plummeting into the abyss of the cliff below.

With their hearts in their mouth, they dawdle through the relentless fog. They know they are on the right road, but Tim's verdict on this part of the journey is that it's "quite concerning".

In the far distance, they notice a hazy light, suspended in the air like the luminescent fin ray of an anglerfish.

'I wonder what that light is?' Tim ponders aloud.

'I don't know. Maybe it's from a hotel in the distance,' suggests Don.

Curiosity piqued, Tim rolls down the window and sticks his head outside, hoping for a clearer view.

'Oh, it's the moon!' Tim laughs, as the celestial orb becomes apparent behind a hazy cloud, which then clears without warning as they break through the top of the cloud and the fog magically disappears.

'We're here, Dad!' Tim's triumphant voice cuts the silence, as the sat nav confirms their arrival to their overnight camp.
Despite the radiant moonlight, it is pitch-black. They can't see a thing and have to trust the sat nav has guided them to where they should be.

The biting cold prevents them from venturing outside the van or even indulging in a bedtime drink, compelling them to retreat to the warmth of the sleeping bags in their makeshift bed. The chilly summer nights at such high altitudes are unforgiving.

Despite their disorientation, they sleep well, knowing they have parked legally somewhere above the tree line on the Furka Pass, taking advantage of Switzerland's policy on wild camping.

But little did they know that the next morning, a jaw-dropping revelation was about to unfold before their very eyes.

117. AWESOME VISTAS

A breathtaking scene unfolds before them.

Snow-capped mountains, glistening under a clear blue sky, stretch out in front of them, offering stunning panoramic views. The majestic Matterhorn, a magnificent mountain located 50 miles in the distance near the Italian border, is standing tall and proud.

They had no idea this remarkable vista was before them when they had parked up the night before.

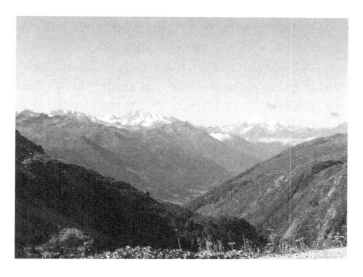

What a view to wake up to.

Overwhelmed by the sheer beauty surrounding them, unwilling to tear themselves away, they take joy in a cup of coffee outside the cafe nearby, savouring the moment. Although Costa has not yet reached the Furka Pass, at least there's an accessible toilet at the Glacier Grotto Shop—very handy for Don.

The Furka Pass is one of the highest mountain passes in Switzerland at nearly 8000 feet - it's over twice the height of Snowdon and almost twice the height of Ben Nevis. Its lofty elevation causes it to be closed from late October until the end of May because of impassable snow.

There are 12 hairpin bends on the Furka Pass and it's a fantastic cycle experience - if a little hairy at times - with only small concrete posts to stop you from going over the edge.

The Pass existed since the 14th century, but they didn't build the road until 1867, when it became the longest pass in Switzerland. Once completed, hotels sprang up along its route - the most spectacular of which was the Belvédère Hotel, built inside the apex of one of the hairpin bends to take advantage of the glorious scenic views down the Rhone Valley. It was built in 1882 and served as a base for exploring the Rhone Glacier.

Sadly, after the 1960s, the demand for an overnight stay there fell away. The hotel slipped into decline and closed in 2015. How sad. Nowhere else in the Alps but at the Belvédère Hotel could guests spend the night at such high altitude and in the morning open the curtains to be greeted by the spectacular view.

The River Rhone cycle route starts at the Rhone Glacier, which moves 30-40 meters a year. Visitors can explore the 100-meter-long tunnel and ice chamber starting in June when the road opens.

How do you stop a glacier from melting? Why, cover it in blankets, of course. During the hot summers, a team places white UV protective sheets over some five acres at the end of the glacier, reflecting the sun's rays and slowing the rate of melting. According to reports, it has an efficiency rate of 70%, offering a glimmer of hope in preserving this natural wonder.

It was Queen Victoria who helped tourism take off on the

Furka Pass when, in 1868, she stayed for four days at the Hotel Furka in Oberwald, high in the mountains.

The Queen wanted to see the Alps because her late husband had told her how beautiful they were, and her doctors also advised that the fresh air would benefit her health.

So, on 22 August 1868, the royal party made an expedition to the Alps and stayed at the Hotel Furka, making daily trips to local beauty spots. In her diary, Queen Victoria described the hotel as a "desolate little house" where, although she enjoyed the mountain scenery during the day, she froze at night. But despite the Queen not raving about her stay at the Hotel Furka, her visit raised the profile of this part of the world, and the Furka Pass rapidly appeared in all the travel guides, drawing more and more tourists year after year.

The Furka Pass gained its fame, however, when the Bond movie *Goldfinger* was filmed there. But in Don's opinion, riding down the Furka Pass on a handcycle is much more fun than driving down in an Aston Martin DB5. You have the wind in your face, you're closer to the tarmac and 46mph seems like 100mph with the handcycle shaking, the wheelchair shaking, and Don shaking.

And so they set off down the Furka Pass as Don rattles along on his handcycle, Tim following part of the way in the van to the next base camp. Then, cycling together, they reach speeds of 62 kilometres per hour while descending, Don out in front, Tim not far behind, stopping only for the occasion *Radler*. Of course!

Then Don, merrily cruising along at over 60 kph, comes to a fork in the road. Not knowing which fork to take, he stops.

Tim doesn't.

There's not enough distance between them to prevent Tim from crashing into Don, as the fork on Tim's wheel - as if emphasising the crash like a pun - hits the hand rim of Don's wheelchair, denting it badly.

Fortunately, the damage is cosmetic, and, checking their maps, they continue on their way.

After some 70 miles, the river has to make a sharp right turn because of the mountains, and after camping overnight near the Swiss town of Sion, they enjoy the ride of their lives, ending up cycling along Lake Geneva.

Then they stop in their tracks at a spellbinding sight ahead.

118. WATER WATER EVERYWHERE...

An enormous jet of water, hundreds of feet high, is squirting up into the air.

It's Geneva's most famous landmark - the Jet d'Eau - installed in 1886 and sited where Lake Geneva exits as the River Rhône.

Visible throughout the city, five hundred litres of water per second are jetted to a height of 476 ft. It's reputedly the world's tallest fountain, an awesome spectacle. At a cost of nearly half a million pounds per year to run, the water shoots from the 4-inch wide nozzle at a mind-blowing speed of over 124 miles an hour. There are approximately 7,000 litres of water in the air at any given moment. You can see it up close if you walk along a stone jetty from the left bank of the lake - though you might get drenched if there's a slight change in wind direction!

After an overnight camp in Geneva, Don and Tim enjoy a relaxing day sightseeing, savouring the sights and sounds of this wonderful city.

They then drive to their new overnight camp at Chanaz planning to take the train back to Geneva the following morning, relishing a cycle ride along the Rhone.

But they hit a problem.

119. IT'S CURTAINS

As they are cycling from Geneva back to Chanaz, the bearing case in Tim's rear wheel surrounding the spindle bursts, causing the bearings to spill out.

Out of the blue, a young cyclist magically appears by Tim's side and speaks to him in French.

Tim, who can't understand a word he's said, answers him in English.

'I think my bearings have gone.'

The young man responds in English, offering to help, effortlessly gliding from one language to the other.

There is a genuine camaraderie among cyclists and this young man - Zhong Lin - having seen Tim's predicament, stops and spends a considerable amount of time attempting to fix the problem.

But the damage is irreparable.

Zhong's caring and considerate support is invaluable to Don and Tim. Speaking fluent French, he books two trains with wheelchair access that enable them to get back to their campsite in Chanaz. Without his assistance, they would have been stranded for hours.

The breakdown happened on Sunday. All French cycle repair shops are closed on both Sunday and Monday. Even if they had waited until Tuesday, they may not have had parts or been able to repair Tim's bike. So with great regret, they cut short their cycle ride and returned home the following day, having cycled a distance of 263 miles along the River Rhone Valley.

It was an incredible journey which they would love to do again.

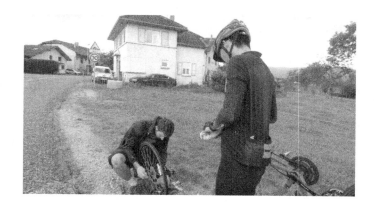

Zhong Lin helping Tim

Don and Tim's verdict of disabled facilities in Austria and Switzerland was a mixed bag. The accessible toilets in Austria were second to none and the best Don had ever encountered anywhere, but his brush with a grumpy Austrian train manager was not an isolated case—it happened several times.

It was a similar story in Switzerland at the rural stations where the platform was lower than the train. At one Swiss rural station, the manager refused point-blank to assist Don off the train. Don had to wedge himself between the doors to prevent the train from moving off, and in the end, a bunch of strangers lifted him down. On the plus side, in the built-up areas, accessibility on Swiss trains was tip-top where the access to the train was the same level as the platform—Don could wheel himself straight on and off without the need for any assistance whatsoever.

Mind you, it's not just abroad Don has experienced unhelpful attitudes on public transport. He might have travelled from Cannes to the Caribbean with no problem—but can he get on a bus in Devon?

Several local bus drivers have grudgingly assisted Don making their displeasure known while unfolding the step for him to board the vehicle. One even refused to allow him onto the bus and drove off, leaving Don to wait another 30 minutes for the next one.

And it's not only drivers either. Belligerent parents on buses can be unforgiving. Often a pushchair will be in the accessible space, but will the parent fold it up to allow Don on the bus? Nope, they will not. Don then has to wait for the next one.

One parent put his fist in Don's face after Don politely suggested if it might be possible to fold up the pushchair and hold the child on his lap, allowing Don into the accessible space. It was an unpleasant exchange, with much foul language from the father of the child, and the bus driver did nothing to help, afraid to interfere with the aggressive parent. The bus was full of passengers who all looked on, helpless. In the end, Don announced he would get off the bus—not to please the abusive parent, but for all the other passengers, not wanting the debacle to hold the bus up any longer.

As for cruise ships, most of them are way ahead of the game when it comes to not only accessibility but also the attitude of staff towards disabled guests. Nothing is too much trouble for them.

But difficulties which are out of the control of the crew can arise at some of the ports—especially if passengers have to use a tender. For wheelchair users, having to board a tender poses extra hazards, and often means missing out altogether on a visit to the port.

Even at ports where the ship can dock, disembarking can be unpredictable. What do you do if you're at the top of a steep gangplank, have mobility issues and suffer from vertigo?

It happened to Don once. The look on Don's face said it all as a high tide in one of the ports we visited affected the gradient of the gangplank down to the quay.

The slope was monumental.

He insisted on going down the ramp backwards. Three

wonderful crew members assisted him—and it wasn't easy for them, but they never gave up and all was well in the end.

So, despite the progress of rights for disabled people, they still often face difficulties, discrimination or unhelpful attitudes. Don has experienced the polarity of human kindness and human grumpiness when it comes to being a wheelchair user, though he's the first to say that on the whole, people are considerate and helpful—a delight to meet. But there's always one. Isn't there?

120. ENABLERS – THE SKY'S THE LIMIT

Despite his disability, Don loves to try various sports. He plays wheelchair tennis, wheelchair basketball and sails with Dart Sailabilty and the Disabled Sailing Association in Torquay. He completed his RYA Powerboat Stage 2 Certificate at the age of 77. He does all he can with the limitations he faces, and with the combination of his can-do attitude and his outgoing personality, he doesn't let his disability prevent him from trying new things.

Organisations that support disabled people in sports and activities deserve high commendation for the sense of achievement they provide to all the disabled (or rather enabled) people they empower to enjoy life to the fullest extent. They recognise that disability is a difference—not a disease. This is key to the ethos they embrace.

There is hardly a sport that disabled people cannot take part in, thanks to the generosity and passion of people who make this happen. Windsurfing, flying aircraft, paragliding, diving, skiing, para-surfing, wheelchair tennis and wheelchair rugby...the list goes on. And I find watching disabled people excel at these sports is just as exciting as watching non-disabled people.

One of our friends, Andy Guy, is a remarkable example of how wheelchair users can excel at extreme sports, and his achievements have taken him all over the world to compete in competitions. He's a world championship medalist in para surfing. He's competed for Great Britain in para table tennis around Europe, and he plays wheelchair rugby in national tournaments throughout the year.

Andy recently posted on Facebook about his journey, and it so eloquently sums up that, with the fusion of drive and determination of both the enabled and the enablers, the sky is the limit -

"Today marks 10 years since I broke my neck flying my kite surfer. Whilst my life was turned upside down and a lot of doors closed to me, a lot more opened. I feel blessed as I look back at all the experiences I've had and all the people I've met because of them! Looking forward to the next 10!"

Finally, there might be a sequel to this book written by Don. Well, he has the title at least: *"Coping with a Crazy Carer."*
Now, that *would* be interesting!

POSTSCRIPT

I'd like to say that I wrote this book out of a motive to encourage disabled people to travel - though the book is probably more about how *not* to travel as a disabled person - especially with a clumsy carer!

Don has many disabled friends who travel the world doing amazing things such as surfing, sailing, skiing, and paragliding. There must be a myriad of handbooks and memoirs on how to travel well as a disabled person, and this isn't it. Mind you, I hope it demonstrates that even the most reticent disabled traveller can nurture the desire to venture abroad.

The inspiration to write this travel memoir came from reading other people's travel memoirs, which I acquired through the "We Love Memoirs" Facebook Group. Admittedly, their memoirs are about amazing travels to exotic places, doing exciting things, and often undertaking extreme sports and activities, or emigrating from the UK to a new life abroad. I confess I began to suffer somewhat from FOMO (fear of missing out) as I read about these adventures in foreign countries. I'd never be able to do anything like that. I've been nowhere and done nothing! ...But then...

Then, quite suddenly, memories of my travels began to surface.

A memory here.

A memory there.

I sought out our photo albums, my travel notes, and other travel memorabilia, and realised that I, too, had some travel stories to share.

I concede our travels might not exactly encompass "globetrotting" given its full meaning, but to us "staycationers", we certainly feel we have trotted a large part of the globe, visiting places we could only ever dream about.

What a privilege it has been to do that.

GLOSSARY

Bally - UK old-fashioned term used instead of a rude word such as "bloody".

Cock-a-hoop - UK term meaning to be extremely happy about something.

Love a duck - UK term: an exclamation of surprise, shock or frustration.

Pigged off - UK term meaning to be annoyed or irritated by something.

Stone the crows - Australian term: an exclamation of incredulity or annoyance.

Suss out - UK informal term meaning to find or discover something.

Tanty - Australian informal term for an outburst of bad temper.

To boot - UK old-fashioned term meaning "also" or "moreover".

ACKNOWLEDGEMENT

I could not have written this memoir without my husband Don, and so my thanks go to him for allowing me to write about him, his disability issues, and his travels as a disabled (differently-abled) person. Also my thanks go to Tim, our son, and his continuing care and support.

Huge thanks to my dream team of BETA readers: Pat Ellis, Julie Haigh, Beth Haslam, Rebecca Hislop, Valerie Poore, Simon Michael Prior, Alison Ripley Cubitt, and Alyson Sheldrake. Their hard work, patient support, encouragement and constructive criticism have been invaluable to me.

My heartfelt thanks to Maggie Raynor for her super artwork for the cover, capturing the title so well, and to Ant Press for formatting the cover. I'm very grateful.

My thanks also go to the Ballard family for the use of the cartoon by Jeremy Ballard of Simon Rattle in Spain.

My thanks to Andy Guy, for permitting me to quote his Facebook post.

ABOUT THE AUTHOR

Dawn Fallon

Dawn Fallon was born in Birmingham in 1959. After studying music she graduated in 1980 but laid aside her musical ambitions when she entered the Civil Service. She met Don in 1992 and moved to Devon when they married in 1994. They have one son, Tim.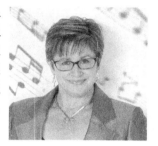

BOOKS BY THIS AUTHOR

Confessions Of A Vat Inspector

A memoir detailing the author's work as a VAT Control Officer in HM Customs & Excise during the late 80s and early 90s, visiting businesses in and around Birmingham to inspect their accounts for Value Added Tax purposes. The job brings her into contact with some bizarre situations and an interesting variety of business people.

Sam - The Busker's Dog

A dog memoir written in the dog's voice. Sam - the author's adorable Cavalier King Charles Spaniel - writes in detail about his life with the Fallons, including escapades with Don busking out on the streets of Devon.

Diary Of An Able Seaman - 1954: Life Onboard Hms Warrior (R31)

The author's father - Les Smith - kept a diary during his 1954 trip around the Med aboard the aircraft carrier HMS Warrior. Dawn has published his diary, illustrated with many pictures, including Operation Passage to Freedom which evacuated non-Communist refugees from Haiphong.

MESSAGE FROM
THE AUTHOR

Thank you for taking the time to read this memoir. If you enjoyed reading this book as much as I have enjoyed writing it, I would be very much obliged if you could leave a review on Amazon.

Even if you didn't buy the book from Amazon, you can still leave a review there if you have a valid Amazon account - reviews help authors enormously and I read every one with interest and gratitude.

I also have an author page on Facebook, and am on X and Instagram plus I have a YouTube Channel - I'd love to hear from you if you'd like to get in touch.

More Photos of Our Travels

I have an author Blog which has extra photos of our travels, and of Don and Tim and their exploits - https://dawnfallonauthor.blogspot.com

We Love Memoirs!

...and finally, if you love reading memoirs, please do join the wonderful We Love Memoirs community on Facebook. You can chat with the author and other memoir authors and readers by joining this fun and friendly Facebook group
https://www.facebook.com/groups/welovememoirs/

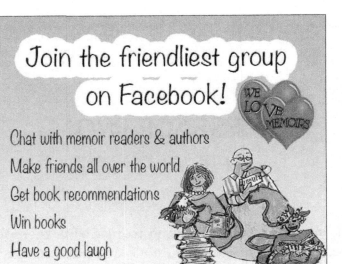

336

Printed in Great Britain
by Amazon

46437093R00195